# Cancer Treatment Breakthroughs

## Milestones, lessons and inspiration for patients, family, friends and survivors

**TIM LADHAMS AND JACKEY COYLE**

Published by Wilkinson Publishing Pty Ltd
ACN 006 042 173
PO Box 24135, Melbourne, VIC 3001, Australia
Ph: +61 3 9654 5446
enquiries@wilkinsonpublishing.com.au
www.wilkinsonpublishing.com.au

Design by Tango Media.
Printed and bound in Australia by Ligare Pty Ltd.

ISBN: 9781925927825

A catalogue record for this book is available from the National Library of Australia

Follow Wilkinson Publishing on social media.

WilkinsonPublishing

wilkinsonpublishinghouse

WPBooks

*Cancer Treatment Breakthroughs* is a book that I would love to have had 20 years ago when I was diagnosed with cancer and felt so overwhelmed and underprepared. Tim Ladhams and Jackey Coyle have created a wonderful book that intelligently melds science, psychology and personal narratives to create a comprehensive overview of the current state of cancer research, medical treatments and management strategies. The manner in which the personal stories are woven throughout the book provides invaluable insights into the lived experiences of cancer sufferers and survivors.

– Dr Sarah Francis, Director, Melbourne Mindfulness Institute

The only book that truly makes sense of the complexities of cancer. Informative, jargon-free and practical.

– Alexandra Stewart, CEO, Centre for Cancer Nutrition

I did not find this a comfortable book to read. And I believe it takes a particular kind of dedication to produce a book such as this.
For some people this is an important and necessary contribution. It could lead to decisions and activities that will save lives. This book does not set out to be an encyclopaedia of cancer, but it is in some ways. I don't believe that this is a book to just dip into. We learn that an early lump or tumour is not necessarily cancer, unless it continues, or changes to some other place. While warning that there are many kinds of cancer, the opening chapter does list the most well-known and most feared. Each subsequent chapter begins with a well-written story of a cancer sufferer's journey, and it is told in a clear way which enables the reader possibly to identify with this experience. But the heart of this book seems to be in the medical procedures: surgery, radiotherapy, chemotherapy, immunotherapy and combination of treatments.

This book strikes a remarkable balance, with the medical procedures incorporating a personal introductive narrative, but then moving into analytical and professor-based details of treatment.

In an age where the media is often distorted by opinion and fake news, here we have a thorough discussion of testing, and many samples, but also the new discoveries, which might make all the difference, but cannot be given immediately to the general public without further careful research. It is logical that this discussion is followed by the question of living life to the full, especially with extended life or full recovery, and the authors have added the need to eat wisely, which they have supported by a large collection of very easy recipes and recommendations.

– Trevor Code

# CONTENTS

# PROLOGUE

I didn't make it back in time. I got to London within thirty hours of receiving the call I had been dreading, knowing it could come at any time, but my father had slipped away.

At least I had a chance to spend some time with him a month and a half before, when I had rushed back from Australia after his cancer had reappeared. I think he knew, when we said goodbye then, that it was for the last time. As I pulled out of the drive he appeared in the spare bedroom window to wave me off, an effort that would have taken up all of the little energy he had by then.

The palliative care nurses had promised me they would try to read the signs and call me in time for me to get back from Melbourne. But they had warned me there was every chance the end would come quickly when it did. Six weeks previously, in August 2009, the nurses hadn't known how long he had, but for Father's sake it was a case of the sooner the better. He would only have got weaker, there would have come a stage when my mother wouldn't be able to cope looking after him at home, and he would have had to have gone to a hospice. That he was still at home when the time came, looking out over his beloved Marlborough Downs through his bedroom window, was a blessing.

The initial prognosis had been positive. The specialist believed he had caught it early, and proclaimed the February 2008 operation to remove the oesophageal cancer a success. In July that year he had seemed to be on the mend. My wife and I went over and Father took us and my mother on a road trip around the south-west of England. He was still very thin, but eating more and more and enjoying his real ale again. Twelve months later, however, the reflux returned, and he started to struggle to eat and drink. A tiny bit of the cancer had evidently survived the treatment and had made into the lymph node, from where it spread rapidly. No new chemotherapy, nor a second operation, would have been of any use. At that point, there was nothing that could be done.

The whole family was in a state of shock when Father was diagnosed, and in the months that followed we went through a roller-coaster of emotions. We put our faith in the medical professionals, were overjoyed in the days after the operation when it was deemed a success, hoped beyond hope that the cancer wouldn't return, then sat by helplessly when it did so.

Father was stoic in the face of the prognosis when the cancer returned—this encouraged us to try and deal with the situation. We put all our efforts into improving his quality of life in the time he had left by doing practical things: moving more furniture and lots of books into his room, organising palliative care nurse visits and trying to be cheerful around him. All the time, however, there was the knowledge that it was ultimately all in vain.

Since then, I have asked myself so many questions. I didn't really even understand what cancer was. What caused him to get this form of cancer in the first place? Would the outcome have been different if the cancer had been caught earlier? Would there have been a different outcome if he was diagnosed today? What is being done to try and ensure as few people, and their families, as possible have to go through what we went through? Will cancer ever actually be beaten in the future?

*Tim Ladhams*

◆ ◆ ◆

Rebecca looked tired and drawn. But that was nothing new—she had always given 150%, whether caring for her husband and daughters, staying in touch with our parents and siblings, or lecturing, mentoring, researching and writing at university.

It was late 2011. We had met for coffee in a Flinders Lane cafe. Rebecca was just back from a trip to North America so I was expecting lots of news and photos. Then I'd show her around the hottest new shops and bars in town. We'd shared a love of Melbourne style ever since we'd lived and worked together, tailoring clothes in my shop. Later she moved to north-eastern New South Wales and we collaborated on music research.

We didn't end up looking at photos or going shopping. Rebecca broke her news: she had been diagnosed with cancer of the bowel. The symptoms had begun to show up before travelling, but she had been caught up with preparations and left it until her return to get checked out. She found the travel arduous, and struggled to fulfil what she had aimed to do. The cancer had metastasised to her liver by now.

I was struggling to take in Rebecca's soft words amid the clatter of the cafe. We had no experience of cancer in our family. I had no idea what to expect. What could I do to help my little sister? I had always been able to, when she needed it.

I spent the next year running up frequent flyer points visiting the Northern Rivers, sitting with her as the icy chemo drugs coursed through her body, trying to make it possible for her to rest. Midyear, we visited the Australian Broadcasting Corporation Lismore studio to talk about the music we had researched. In early November, she rang me during a gig at the Wangaratta Festival of Jazz. She was going into palliative care.

The last thing she would ask of me: to let our parents and siblings know. My parents were not well enough to fly so I promised to be with her for them. My sisters flew from overseas, but only one made it in time.

Rebecca wasn't speaking any more. She lay still, her hand positioned perfectly to receive mine. The hospice room was tranquil, fragrant with blooms, as she faded. She was only 56 when she died in November 2012.

Seven years later, the grief returned when my husband Jules tested positive—first for a bowel-cancer screening, and then for a substantially sized tumour. Was it benign or malignant? What was lurking underneath? Even the doctors didn't know. We put everything on hold as we waited for certainty.

Jules underwent major surgery and, as he began to recover, we awaited the results of yet more pathology tests.

Miraculously, no cancer had remained. He is now fully recovered, with no need for further investigations.

People sometimes object to being invited to participate in Australia's bowel-cancer-screening program. Jules had complained, too. My response remains the same: 'Just do it'. Nothing will bring back Rebecca, but early detection saved Jules.

*Jackey Coyle*

◆ ◆ ◆

The very word *cancer* strikes fear into the hearts of most people.

Like us, the people we spoke to for this book each have their own cancer journey, whether as a researcher, doctor or patient. We have gathered together a wealth of information so you will understand more about the disease, the treatments and staying well afterwards.

Australia consistently figures in the top countries in the world for early detection and excellent treatment. While we suffer high levels of certain types of cancers, such as skin, prostate, lung, bowel and breast, we have the lowest cancer mortality rate in the world. Our policy and planning infrastructure within our healthcare system comes out on top globally.

In the pages that follow we will look at the latest developments in every facet of cancer treatment. We'll learn about advanced diagnostic techniques that are able to detect cancer earlier than ever before in its progress. We'll look at the latest developments in the longstanding methods of treating cancer, and we'll learn about fundamentally new approaches that are revolutionising the treatment of cancer.

We'll investigate the most important new therapies that are now available to treat the most common forms of cancer that afflict millions of people around the world, and see what is being done to broaden our understanding of the rarer forms of the disease, which to date have been so difficult to treat.

In the process, we will meet a number of cancer patients who have recently undergone some of the breakthrough forms of treatment being covered. We will learn about their cancer journeys, the impact the disease has had on their lives and those of their families, and find out about their experiences of the treatments they have had and their outcomes.

Finally, we'll establish if there are any ways we can improve our chances of surviving cancer through lifestyle choices—thinking carefully about what we eat, ensuring we stay as active as possible, getting enough sleep, and having a positive mindset—if we suffer the misfortune of contracting one of the many different forms of the disease. We will also give some tips for survivors, as well as supporting someone with cancer, and finally some simple recipes to get the most out of every bite we eat.

# Chapter 1

# THE WORLD'S BIGGEST PROBLEM

Cancer is manifesting at an ever-increasing rate, and predictions are that the world will see more than 20 million cases a year within the next two decades. Alongside the human cost is an enormous economic impact.

In this chapter we will delve into exactly what we're looking at:

◆ what cancer is

◆ how and why people develop it

◆ how cancer treatment evolved through the millennia

◆ the astounding treatment breakthroughs we will be covering later.

Let's begin with some facts and figures. More than 200 different cancers have been identified to date, with more coming to light all the time. In 2020, the latest year for which the World Health Organization's (WHO) International Agency for Research on Cancer has collated figures, almost 10 million deaths were attributed to cancer in all its forms and 19 million new cases of cancer were diagnosed. The incidence of the condition in all its manifestations has increased by a third since the 1970s, and the agency's forecasts predict that the number of newly diagnosed cases per year will rise to over 30 million globally in 2040. Alongside the human cost is an enormous economic impact, with the latest WHO data estimating cancer's total economic cost at over USD 1.16 trillion per annum.

This increase in cancer occurrence is resulting in a greater focus on understanding and treating this growing problem. Today in the United States alone, the federal budget allocates around USD 6 billion a year to the National Cancer Institute for research into cancer and its treatment. This figure does not include charitable donations or private funding. Cancer Research UK has almost 4000 full-time employees and 40,000 volunteers, and in 2012 spent GBP 100 million developing Europe's largest biomedical research facility, the Francis Crick Institute. In Australia, where one in two men and one in three women will be diagnosed with cancer by the age of 85, over 20% of all health research expenditure is targeted at cancer. The direct cost of cancer to the Australian health system stands at over $6 billion.

These are enormous sums of money being spent on the diagnosis and treatment of cancer, and research into it, for wealthy first-world nations. So how do developing countries cope? The reality is that their more meagre resources mean a heavier toll. Over 70% of cancer deaths globally today take place in low- and middle-income nations. In 2017 only 26% of low-income countries provided cancer pathology services in their public health sectors.

## IT'S ALL ABOUT CELLS

So, just what is this scourge?

Cancer is a genetic mutation of cells in any part of the body. Healthy cells grow and divide in a controlled way, then become dormant and eventually die, to be replaced by new ones. A cell's DNA governs how it acts; if it becomes damaged, this process is interrupted. The cell grows and divides repeatedly and uncontrollably, and continues to do so rather than dying out.

The uncontrollable growth produces cells that all have the same abnormal DNA as the original bad cell. The group of cancerous cells that affect the organ or part of the body in which they originated is known as a *primary growth* or *tumour*, and is also referred to as *localised cancer*.

The body creates new blood vessels through a process called *angiogenesis*. This process is beneficial when the body uses it to repair scar tissue and to support the embryo during pregnancy, but it feeds tumours and enables them to grow. As a cancer tumour grows it damages the surrounding tissue, interfering with the digestive, nervous and circulatory systems.

Cancers can spread via membranes, the lymph nodes or bloodstream to create secondary tumours in other parts of the body, a process known as *metastasis*. These cancers, described as *invasive cancers*, are harder to treat than primary tumours, and account for 90% of all cancer deaths.

Malignant cells are liable to spread from their original position in the body because they are more agile than healthy ones—a breakdown in their molecular structure enables them to detach themselves from their usual position and to get through smaller gaps than normal cells. This allows them to break through membranes that line structures in the body, usually keeping groups of cells in different parts of the body apart.

Tumours are fed by blood vessels and cells that detach into those vessels can then be carried into the circulatory system carrying blood around the body. Such cells can travel a long way from their original source, until they get stuck in smaller vessels and start to grow in their new location. Tumours that spread this way are known as *circulating tumour cells*.

Cancer cells can also spread from their original site via the lymphatic system. Lymph vessels spread out from nodes and act as a filter, carrying immune cells that attack infections. Tumour cells can detach and get into the lymph vessels, which act as an alternative transport system to blood circulation. In this way they can carry tumour cells to new areas of the body, different from those in which they formed. The immune cells are not always capable of killing the cancer cells within them, and this can lead to the cells forming secondary tumours.

## Types of cancer

Cancers are usually named for the organ or cell type of the primary cancer, even if they spread to other parts of the body. For example, a cancer that begins in the lungs and spreads to the liver is still called lung cancer. There are broad categories for different types of cancer:

**Carcinoma**: a cancer that starts in the skin or the tissues that line or cover organs, e.g. melanoma

**Central nervous system cancer**: cancer that begins in the brain or spinal cord, e.g. glioma

**Leukaemia**: cancer that begins in the tissues that make blood cells, such as the bone marrow

**Lymphoma** and **myeloma**: cancers of the immune system, e.g. Hodgkin lymphoma

**Sarcoma**: cancer that begins in bone, fat, muscle, blood vessel, or other supportive or connective tissue, e.g. osteosarcoma

## WILL I GET IT?

Many different factors increase the risk of cancer. Some may be unavoidable; some you can affect by modifying your behaviour or environment.

On the unavoidable side, some cancers are inherited, passed from one generation of a family to the next genetically. The other unavoidable risk factor we are all vulnerable to, irrespective of lifestyle choices or where and how we are brought up, is ageing—as we get older, the number of potentially malignant mutations of our DNA increases.

Other risks are posed by a person's lifestyle or environment. In developed countries key risk factors in the growing number of cancer sufferers are tobacco use, alcohol use, unhealthy diet and lack of physical activity, despite our increased awareness of these risks.

In the developing world, the most common causes of the condition are chronic infections—particularly hepatitis—and air pollution.

Governments and health agencies are struggling to cope with the proliferation of cancers in many of the world's poorest countries, due to both financial constraints and the 'brain drain' that sees some of the best-credentialed researchers and medical professionals leaving low- and middle-income nations for the US, Europe and the world's other wealthiest countries.

## CANCER ACROSS THE MILLENNIA

The term *cancer* was first coined by Hippocrates—the 'father of medicine'—around 400 BCE. Ever since then mankind has been looking for a cure. Another Greek physician Galen (130–200 CE) used the Greek word *oncos,* meaning swellings, to describe tumours—from him we have adopted the term *oncology* to refer to cancer-related topics.

In most cases cancer returned after tumours were removed surgically, resulting in the belief that it was incurable. Since primitive operations caused severe blood loss, intense pain, infections and other complications after the procedure, the general approach for the best part of 2000 years was to manage cancer rather than attempt to treat it.

In the 17th century a belief spread throughout Europe that cancer was contagious. Cancer hospitals were built in isolated locations for fear that patients would infect the populations in towns and cities. Scottish surgeon John Hunter contributed greatly to the development of more precise surgery in the 18th century. He successfully removed primary tumours, and his observations about secondary tumours proved to be the bedrock that enabled the theory of metastasis to later be founded.

A century later the discovery of anaesthesia precipitated a huge advance in the development of surgery. William Halsted performed the first radical mastectomy in 1882, significantly improving the outlook for breast cancer patients in the United States. Halsted, William Handley in the UK and Theodor Billroth in Austria pioneered surgery to remove the lymph nodes adjoining tumours as well as the tumours themselves, a development that in many cases reduces the risk of the cancer returning.

Also in the 19th century, pathology was developed, thanks mainly to improvements in microscopic technology. Now surgeons had a better idea of whether or not they had successfully removed all the cancer using these new surgical procedures.

Radiotherapy was used to treat cancer patients for the first time in the last few years of the 1800s, and chemotherapy arose as a result of research into chemical agents during World War II. The first screening technique to come into widespread use was the Pap test in the 1960s, cutting the mortality rate among cervical cancer sufferers by approximately 70%. The mammogram was promoted as a means of early detection of breast cancer in the second half of the 1970s.

## NEW APPROACHES

Mortality rates around the world continued to rise all the way up until the late 20th century, despite these developments in surgery, anaesthesia, therapy and screening. Death rates did begin to fall in the early 1990s, but there can be no doubt that now—in the third decade of the 21st century—new breakthroughs in cancer treatment are being made at a higher rate than ever before.

We now have a better understanding of the biology of cancer, with new technology that was unimaginable a century ago. Different branches of the medical profession are collaborating with one another, blowing apart the silos that previously inhibited the sharing of knowledge.

Despite the fact that cancer in all its forms claimed the lives of approximately ten million people around the world in 2020, the chances of surviving cancer are now better than at any time in the past. Huge research budgets and the application of science and technology have increased our understanding of cancer, and how it can be better countered. In the last 40 years cancer survival rates have doubled, and today half of those diagnosed with cancer survive for at least ten years.

Until the early years of this century there were fundamentally three main fields of cancer treatment—surgery, chemotherapy and radiotherapy. Today, however, we are seeing not only advances in these areas, but also brand-new approaches to cancer treatment.

Research—into our childhood environment, our lifestyle, our fundamental genetic make-up and our immune systems—is expanding not only the way we look at cancer, but also the number of fronts we can fight it on. A recent marked increase in collaboration between cancer specialists around the world means globally coordinated research projects give more comprehensive results—due to the greater number of patients involved—more quickly. This in turn means that technologies, medicines and combinations of types of treatment that prove successful can be made available sooner than studies from single centres, and trials run out of individual hospitals or laboratories.

A UK project has mapped the DNA of over 85,000 people—drawn from patients with rare diseases, cancer patients, and the families of those patients—in an attempt to develop more targeted treatment. By taking the data from three cells of cancer patients—one from a healthy cell inside a tumour, once from a cancerous cell within the same tumour and a third from the blood—the researchers are building a better understanding of an individual's vulnerability to specific diseases. This will help them develop ways of making earlier diagnoses of these conditions. And for the patients taking part in the project, the data are providing a greater understanding of which type of treatment might be most suitable for them. The project is being expanded with the aim of getting the data of ten times as many people by 2023. This form of research, *genome mapping*, can be described as 'going on a journey with a far more detailed map than was previously available, and makes it far more likely we'll reach our destination'.

Immunotherapy is now in the vanguard of the fight against many forms of cancer. *Science* magazine, one of the world's foremost scientific journals, nominated cancer immunotherapy as its 2013 breakthrough. At the time, the panel who made the decision admitted they had agonised over it because of the very small number of patients who had been able to benefit from it at such an early stage in its development. Since the article was published, numerous clinical trial results have supported its assertion that immunotherapy is a 'turning point' in the fight against cancer. In a UCLA study completed in 2019, the immunotherapy drug pembrolizumab helped more than 15% of people with advanced non-small cell lung cancer live for at least five years. Immunotherapy uses substances naturally produced in the body, rather than chemically-produced drugs, to boost our natural immune system so it can identify, target and attack cancer cells.

These breakthroughs are just a couple of examples of the revolution in cancer treatment in the last decade—we will now look closely at all the latest key advances in the diagnosis and treatment of cancer.

Chapter 2

# WHAT ARE WE DEALING WITH HERE? ADVANCED DIAGNOSTICS

The treatment breakthroughs covered in this book are having some success against advanced stage cancers. Nevertheless, the chances of survival are greatly improved the earlier the cancer is detected. In this chapter, we will look at diagnostics in all their forms:

◆ how nuclear medicine is helping early diagnosis

◆ how doctors diagnose the 'big five' cancers

◆ how tests are becoming simple and cost effective enough for a GP's surgery.

Before we look into the various ways the medical profession diagnoses cancer, we'll find out how identifying a tumour very early in its development has allowed Malcolm to carry on living life to the full.

## Catching it early

Malcolm is a fit and active Queenslander in his mid-60s who spends his life on his feet, renovating houses from Monday to Friday and enjoying his weekends on the tennis court.

A few years ago Malcolm started to feel uncomfortable after meals. Increasingly frequent bouts of heartburn and bloating persuaded him to go to his GP. After a series of tests and visits to different specialists, Malcolm learned he had developed coeliac disease.

Finding out what was causing the problem and, more importantly, what he could do about it put Malcolm back on track. He took advice, researched the disease and overhauled his diet. Within months the discomfort had disappeared and Malcolm was back to his usual sprightly self.

Malcolm was concerned, therefore, when he woke up one night late in 2020 in severe discomfort. Initially he assumed he had stepped outside his usual careful diet regime—he had been out to dinner with friends—and tried to sleep it off. But the stomach pain increased and he took himself to his local emergency department. Malcolm was given some medicine to ease the discomfort, blood tests were conducted and a computerised tomography (CT) scan performed, but the team was unable to find a cause for the pain. By the morning it had subsided and he was discharged.

Two evenings later the pain returned and Malcolm returned to Emergency. Once again, tests and a scan failed to find the root of the problem. When Malcolm learned he was to be discharged again, he asked for a second opinion and was referred to the Royal Brisbane Hospital. A specialist there took particular interest in the fact that Malcolm had had a number of skin lesions removed over the years. Like all young Queenslanders, Malcolm had spent his childhood out in the sun. He only started wearing a hat and covering up in middle age, as the risk of skin cancer came into public consciousness. Knowing he had potentially put himself in harm's way as a younger man, Malcolm was diligent about checking his skin regularly and making sure anything that appeared was removed promptly. Although all the removed lesions had been checked, with biopsies coming up negative for melanoma, the specialist decided to investigate further.

A magnetic resonance imaging (MRI) scan revealed a tiny mass that was a cause for concern and Malcolm was booked in for a colonoscopy later the same week. A *biopsy*—a detailed look at a sample of tissue taken during the procedure—revealed the presence of cancerous cells. This came as a terrible shock to Malcolm, but the specialist assured him that the size and nature of what he had found indicated that the tumour had only recently developed. Further tests found no evidence that the cancer had spread.

Malcolm embarked on an eight-week course of chemotherapy, involving a few hours at the hospital one day a week. He experienced mild side effects from the chemotherapy and felt 'a bit knocked about' for 48 hours or so after each bout of treatment. He was able to continue working a few days a week, with the discomfort he had experienced before the diagnosis gradually subsiding. At the conclusion of the treatment, an MRI scan revealed that the tumour had shrunk, and he was prescribed an immunotherapy drug that he takes daily.

Six months on from his initial admission to his local emergency department, Malcolm is living life to the full once again. He is more cautious than ever before about what he eats, and keeps to a strict regime of taking his immunotherapy medication. He is working regularly and recently returned to the tennis court. The cause of the cancer is unproven, whether or not it is related to his early years of exposure to the Queensland sun.

Malcolm is looking forward to watching his young grandchildren grow up. He is thankful that the tumour was caught so early, and that he is now able to contemplate getting even stronger.

———————————————————————

Many people do not realise they have cancer for months or even years after it has first developed. In most forms of the disease symptoms do not present until it is well established, and often has already spread from the site of the original tumour. This scenario makes treatment more complicated, and invariably reduces the likelihood that 100% of the cancerous cells can be identified and eliminated.

Therefore, medical researchers are working on a two-pronged approach—while they are putting an enormous effort into developing the way cancer is treated, they are also investigating how more cancers can be detected earlier.

## TAKING SCANS NUCLEAR

Nuclear medicine is responsible for some of the most important advances in diagnosing multiple forms of cancer. Specific tests have also improved the early detection rates for some of the most common forms of cancer that are responsible for most cancer deaths worldwide. In the case of two of these forms—skin and breast cancers—the most effective diagnostic tests are biopsies, which are detailed in Chapter 3, Surgical techniques.

### CT scans

A *computerised tomography* (CT) scan uses multiple X-rays beamed at different angles to build up a 3-D image of the area of the body being investigated. Before the scan, a dye is injected into a vein in the arm. This dye moves through the bloodstream and helps the images of tissue and organs show up more clearly on the scan.

This type of scan is able to pick up smaller tumours than a standard single X-ray—and gives a more accurate idea of the size of any tumour—because it shows depth as well as surface area.

The lymphatic system is the main conduit for the spread of cancer around the body, so a CT scan of the chest area is very important as it will reveal whether any cancer has made its way into the lymph nodes in the chest.

### MRI scans

*Magnetic resonance imaging* (MRI) scans use radio waves to produce images of soft tissue, such as organs and muscles, that X-rays do not pick up. An MRI scan is taken inside a tube, so it produces images from all angles around the body. Because of this, it is adept at identifying tumours that would be hidden by a bone mass or another organ if they were scanned from only a front-on or side-on angle.

MRI scans are most effective in detecting brain tumours, soft tissue sarcomas—cancers that develop in fat, muscles and blood vessels—and tumours in the spinal cord. As well as being used to diagnose cancer, MRI scans are used to look at the extent to which the size of tumours have altered after treatment.

## PET imaging

*Positron emission tomography* (PET) imaging is sensitive enough to detect changes in the chemical make-up of an organ or tissue, even before those changes impact the structure of the affected area. It can detect diseases at a very early stage and help doctors decide on the most effective treatment, or combination of treatments.

The earlier any form of cancer is detected, the better the chances of successful treatment. Larger-than-usual amounts of glucose are a by-product of the formation of a tumour, and therefore strongly indicate cancer in its earliest stages. A PET scan reveals the levels of glucose consumption in cells and can, therefore, aid in the diagnosis of cancer before any symptoms have manifested themselves.

A decade ago almost three-quarters of the $2 trillion spent on health care in the United States went towards treatment of chronic diseases and attempts to deal with conditions in their advanced stages. PET imaging is important in improving survival rates for cancer patients by diagnosing them before their cancer takes hold and spreads.

As a PET scan provides an image of the whole body and is able to differentiate between an active tumour and scar tissue, it is useful in monitoring the spread of cancer. Patients will have scans at regular intervals throughout a course of treatment to see if it is working.

PET scans are invariably carried out in conjunction with a CT scan, which images the structure of bones and tissue. In this way the chemical composition and the physical shape and size of groups of cells can be analysed at the same time.

PET scans involve an injection of a tiny amount of radioactive material; in most scans this material is a biologically active molecule called *fluorodeoxyglucose* (FDG) with a similar structure to sugar. It has minimal side effects, so patients can resume most normal activities immediately afterwards.

## A TARGETED APPROACH

These scans can be used in to diagnose a range of different cancers. Often, however, accurate diagnosis requires specific tests designed to uncover the tell-tale signs unique to the make-up and development of a particular form of the disease.

In 2018 the WHO recorded the highest incidence of new cases of cancer as those affecting the lungs, the breasts, the bowel and the prostate. These four forms of cancer saw over one million recorded cases—lung and breast topped the list with over two million each. We'll now look at recent developments that have helped earlier and/or more accurate diagnosis of these forms of cancer. We'll also look at ovarian cancer, as this form of the disease has until recently been notoriously difficult to diagnose. As ovarian cancer is a particularly aggressive form and the cancer was already at an advanced stage by the time diagnosis was made, survival rates have been lower than most other forms.

### Lung cancer diagnostics

Lung cancer is responsible for more deaths than any other form of the disease. The most widely used diagnostic test for lung cancer is a chest X-ray, but this only identifies tumours that are more than a centimetre wide, meaning they are not caught when they first develop. It can also fail to find tumours that are 'hiding' behind organs in the chest cavity.

A number of tests using a microscopic camera have been developed, which can identify smaller tumours and those in hard-to-reach areas of the lungs.

A *bronchoscopy* is carried out under local anaesthetic, and involves the passing of a very thin tube with a tiny camera through the mouth, down the throat and into the lungs. The tube is designed to carry out two forms of biopsy called *washing* and *brushing*. A drop of fluid is injected and then withdrawn again—washed through it—so the cells of the lungs can be tested. The tube also 'brushes' off cells on the walls of the airways in the lungs so they too can be analysed.

A specialised form of bronchoscopy, *endobronchial ultrasound* (EBUS), uses soundwaves to measure the size of the tumour. A needle can be attached to the end of the tube to take samples from lymph nodes and the tumour itself, a process called *endobronchial ultrasound-guided transbronchial needle aspiration* (EBUS TBNA).

A *thoracoscopy* is a similar process to a bronchoscopy, but the tube is inserted via an incision made between two ribs rather than through the mouth. A *thoracotomy* involves a larger incision being made in the back, to provide access into the chest cavity. The decision as to which of these procedures is most appropriate is governed by where in or around the lungs the tumour, or suspected tumour, is located.

### Breast cancer diagnostics

Cancer cells produce proteins called *antigens* that trigger the body's immune system to produce *antibodies* to fight them, known as *autoantibodies*. At the UK's 2019 National Cancer Research Institute conference, researchers from the University of Nottingham presented the results of the trial of a blood test that successfully diagnosed cases of breast cancer by identifying the presence of these autoantibodies. Having established tumour-associated antigens that are associated with breast cancer, the team were able to detect whether or not there were autoantibodies against them in blood samples taken from patients, matching their samples with those from a control group of people who do not have breast cancer.

The trial identified the antigens in people who had experienced no symptoms of breast cancer, and the team are expanding the trial. They hope the research will result in developing a test that will diagnose breast cancer five years before any symptoms manifest themselves and be available for general use by 2023 or 2024.

### Bowel cancer diagnostics

CT scans, MRI scans and PET scans are all useful tools for staging bowel cancer, and for checking on the progress once treatment has started, but initial diagnosis depends on obtaining a tissue sample from the bowel and analysing it to establish if there are cancerous cells present. The most effective way of obtaining the sample is by performing a colonoscopy.

During a colonoscopy a very thin tube with a microscopic camera on the end is inserted into the bowel through the patient's rectum. The tube is passed through the bowel with specialists studying the image that the camera relays back to their screen. If there are any abnormalities they use a tiny brush attached to the tube to take a sample, which is then removed for analysis in the lab.

### Prostate cancer diagnostics

The most basic tests for prostate cancer are easy to conduct but not definitive. A high level of *prostate-specific antigen* (PSA), a protein that forms in the prostate gland, can be an indicator of prostate cancer. However, PSA is present in both healthy and cancerous cells, and the PSA level can be raised by other factors such as a benign prostate enlargement or an infection. A digital examination of the rectum will fail to pick up very small tumours in their early stages or tumours forming out of reach. New diagnostic methods developed in the last few years have increased the reliability of testing for prostate cancer, and reduced the number of 'false positive' tests and the unnecessary treatment that results.

The Prostate Health Index (PSI) test was approved for use in Europe in 2010 and in the USA and elsewhere around the world soon after that. The PHI still focuses on a patent's PSA, but can identify different forms of the protein and identify whether a raised level is the sign of a benign or malignant condition.

The PCA3 is a gene found in prostate cells that produces a protein. When cancer is present in the prostate it produces increased levels of the PCA3 protein, and when the concentration of the protein reaches an elevated point it leaks into the urine. PCA3 protein levels do not increase in the case of benign conditions such as prostate enlargement, meaning a urine test showing a high PCA3 level is a strong indicator of prostate cancer.

## Ovarian cancer diagnostics

CT and MRI scans are capable of revealing an unidentified mass in the pelvic area, but cannot detect whether or not the mass is cancerous. One test has been devised very recently to diagnose early-stage ovarian cancer, and another gives doctors very good feedback on how treatment is progressing once the disease has been confirmed.

*Fallopian tube lavage* has only been developed in the last few years, but it is proving to be promising in clinical trials taking place in the United States and Europe. The test is important because it is designed to diagnose ovarian cancer at an earlier stage than has previously been possible. Typical symptoms of ovarian cancer such as feeling bloated, heartburn and back pain are common to many conditions and patients do not suspect ovarian cancer until other causes are investigated.

A non-surgical procedure, fallopian tube lavage collects a small amount of fluid from the fallopian tube, which is then analysed by pathologists. Researchers hope it can be refined and simplified so it can be used to test a large percentage of women, and before any symptoms present, in the same way that the Pap smear is used to screen for cervical cancer.

Ovarian cancer usually results in an increased level of a protein called CA 125 in the patient's blood. Other conditions can produce CA 125 so this test is not used in isolation, but it is a useful tool in monitoring the progress of treatment after a positive diagnosis. Once a benchmark level has been taken, ongoing testing helps indicate the effectiveness of treatment—a reduction in the level suggests treatment is working; no change or an increase in the level of CA 125 will often result in a change of approach.

## MAKING IT SIMPLE

The primary focus of research into diagnostics is to find ways of detecting cancer as early as possible. While some advances are in high-tech imaging and surgical procedures involving microscopic instruments, other developments are simple and cost effective.

In 2019 the Cancer Research UK Cambridge Centre launched a clinical trial on the back of the theory that cancer produces chemicals that are detectable on a person's breath. Scientists are establishing benchmarks for the *volatile organic compounds* (VOCs) released on our breath when healthy cells metabolise. Cancer causes cells to metabolise differently, changing the VOCs, and the two-year trial is designed to ascertain if VOCs can be analysed to diagnose different forms of cancer at an early stage of their development. Promising early results hint at the possibility that at some point in the not-too-distant future a simple breathalyser test could be an important weapon in diagnosing cancer.

Most cancers involve cells that circulate in the patient's bloodstream, so scientists expect that the theory behind the blood test for breast cancer, which we mentioned earlier in this chapter, will work for other forms of the disease. A team from Johns Hopkins University in Baltimore has developed a blood test that measures proteins and tumour-specific mutations in DNA found in the bloodstream. Early results of the trial, published in *Science* magazine, saw the successful detection of eight common forms of cancer. The research is expected to result in straightforward blood tests that accurately diagnose at least some cancers being available in GP surgeries within two to three years.

Chapter 3

# THE CUTTING EDGE SURGICAL TECHNIQUES

Surgery is the oldest form of cancer treatment, but technological innovations have kept it at the forefront of the fight. In this chapter we will reveal:

◆ techniques used for removing tumours

◆ surgery as a diagnostic tool

◆ proactive minimisation of risk

◆ symptom management.

But first, let's look at a keyhole surgery success story.

## Surgery through the keyhole

Alistair is an extremely active man who runs his own successful business in Melbourne. His work takes him criss-crossing the city daily, the country regularly and the globe occasionally. Outside work, Alistair is best known around the traps for his aptitude at playing the bagpipes, an enterprise that involves not just musicality but also a high degree of effort and dexterity.

Alastair's hectic schedule has never been an issue for him—in fact he thrives on it—but a few years ago he found himself getting tired during the day and lacking his customary energy. A blood test revealed he had haemochromatosis, an inherited condition that is one of the most common genetic disorders around the world—

approximately one in every 200 people of Northern European descent carries the gene abnormality that puts them at risk of developing it. Haemochromatosis causes sufferers to absorb too much iron from their food. If left untreated the build-up of iron will eventually damage the heart, liver and other organs.

Management for Alistair involved *serial phlebotomy,* or bloodletting. Alistair gave up one pint of his iron-filled blood every week for a year, and the symptoms abated. Alistair thought he'd had his 'big health problem' and that, as long as he stayed fit and active, all would be well.

Soon after his 64th birthday, however, Alistair began to feel some discomfort in his lower back. When this extended to occasional pain when urinating, he went to see his GP. The initial step was testing for PSA, a protein produced in the prostate gland. With Alistair's PSA slightly elevated the results were not dramatic, but a further test was recommended.

The results of Alistair's biopsy were much starker than that first PSA test. His Gleason Score was 8, a high-range reading that means the prostate cells extracted in the biopsy have significantly mutated, indicating aggressive tumour behaviour in Alistair's prostate gland.

Within two months of first experiencing the discomfort, Alistair was in Melbourne's Epworth Hospital preparing for a radical prostatectomy—the removal of the entire prostate gland. He benefited from having the procedure carried out robotically—he was up and about again in half the time it would have taken had he undergone traditional surgery, due to less blood loss and nerve damage resulting from robotic surgery. The size of the tumour was so large that he would have been in hospital for at least a week after a manual procedure, but Alistair was able to go home within four days.

He was able to return to the office soon after the operation, although his working day was punctuated by 20-minute sessions of radiotherapy designed to kill off any cancer cells that had spread beyond his prostate. Now he takes a three-monthly hormone therapy that supplements the effects of the radiation, aiming to reduce the risk of any recurrence of his cancer.

Alistair has to do ongoing physiotherapy to strengthen his pelvic floor, counteracting the side effects of the radiotherapy treatment. He has, however, had no ill effects from the surgery itself, despite it being a major operation. Alistair is adamant that he would not have been able to make anything like this recovery without the unwavering support of his wife and his mates. He is sure that his determination to come through, from his initial diagnosis and throughout treatment, helped him to get that outcome and he would not have been able to keep up that resolve without their encouragement.

The biggest issue Alistair is confronting now is the suspicion aroused by his bagpipes as he plans another overseas trip. Despite having had them since 1957, he still has to submit a mountain of paperwork to customs to get them in and out of the country, as they take a good deal of persuading each time that such an extraordinary-looking contraption is actually a musical instrument!

---

Surgery used to always involve scalpels, and result in lots of stitches and long scars. Today, though, the treatment of cancer uses a host of advanced surgical methods designed to be minimally invasive.

Lasers, high-frequency electrical currents and liquid nitrogen are employed in different procedures to improve effectiveness and make the patient's recovery as quick and painless as possible.

Computer-controlled robotic instruments and surgical microscopes enable surgeons to be more accurate, and to operate in parts of the body that were previously inaccessible or too delicate for surgical procedures. Surgeons can now remove smaller tumours from harder-to-reach locations in the body using laparoscopic and microsurgical instruments, and improvements in imaging have increased the chances of removing all the cancerous material during an operation.

Minimally invasive surgical techniques are reducing the impact surgery has on patients, allowing them to resume a more active life more quickly after their procedure.

## A MORE REFINED APPROACH

The original intention of surgery for cancer patients was to try and remove every cancerous cell from the body. So, in the case of breast cancer, the *radical mastectomy*—removal of the entire breast and the associated lymph nodes under the armpit—was the norm. Surgery itself, however, rarely removed every trace of the cancer and the majority of patients suffered relapses—some within a couple of months of the surgery, others in the years following it.

Throughout the 20th century the more common approach became less invasive surgery, combined with at least one other form of treatment. In the first half of the century, the norm involved more targeted surgery supplemented by radiotherapy, and later doctors usually prescribed chemotherapy and/or radiotherapy as well as an operation. This combination of treatment types meant surgery did not result in the removal of as much tissue as previously.

Improvements in scanning and imaging also allowed cancer to be diagnosed without the need for an exploratory operation. In addition, imaging began to be employed to improve the accuracy of surgery, helping the surgeon to home in on the exact tissue requiring removal, thereby reducing the impact of the procedure on the body.
Surgery can be used to achieve a range of outcomes for cancer patients. Different surgical techniques are used to:

◆ confirm a diagnosis and 'stage' the cancer—assess how far it has spread

◆ remove tissue that has a high risk of being affected by cancer

◆ attempt to cure cancer by removal of the tumour

◆ reduce the size of a tumour that cannot be fully removed so subsequent treatment is more likely to succeed

◆ improve function and/or appearance of a part of the body affected by cancer

◆ reduce pain and ease symptoms arising from cancer.

## *Diagnostic surgery*

The original symptoms of cancer can also be indicative of other, less serious conditions. For example, heartburn can be the result of a reflux disease or asthma, but is also brought on by oesophageal cancer.

Advanced imaging and various tests are able to positively diagnose some cancers, but often a detailed look at a sample of tissue by a pathologist is required to confirm whether a tumour is cancerous. This procedure is called a *biopsy,* and different approaches depend on the location of the tumour:

◆ **Fine needle aspiration** is appropriate for tumours in readily accessible areas of the body. A very thin needle is inserted through the skin into the questionable material and a sample drawn out for testing by pathologists.

◆ **Incisional biopsy** sees part of the tumour removed and examined while the patient is still in theatre, so a larger sample or the whole tumour can be removed at the same time, if that is considered necessary or appropriate.

◆ **Excisional biopsy** involves the whole tumour and a small amount of surrounding healthy tissue being removed. No further treatment may be required if the cancer has not spread and this procedure removes it all. The removal of tissue is guided by a thin tube with a tiny camera. Depending on the location in the body where the tumour is being investigated, the tube may be inserted into one of the body's natural openings such as the mouth (*endoscopic* biopsy), or through an incision made by the surgeon in the patient's abdomen (*laparoscopic* biopsy) or chest (*thoracoscopic* biopsy).

Once cancer is diagnosed, the most urgent task for medical professionals is working out how far advanced the tumour is. The approach to treatment depends on whether or not the cancer has spread from its original site and, if so, where it has spread to. Three measurements are used to classify this staging of cancer—*tumour, node* and *metastasis*—and are referred to using the acronym TNM:

◆ **Tumour**: measured on a scale of 1 to 4, with T1 being a very small tumour and T4 a large one.

◆ **Node**: indicating the number of lymph nodes the cancer has reached. (The lymphatic system is the main conduit of cancer around the body.) This scale goes from N0, showing cancer has not spread to the lymph nodes, to N3 which means the cancer has reached a high number of lymph nodes.

◆ **Metastasis**: gauging whether or not the cancer has spread. A result of M0 means that no other area of the body other than the site of the original tumour has been affected; whereas M1 indicates the cancer has spread to an organ or tissue removed from that site.

Some forms of diagnostic surgery have a *curative* effect, so while they are designed primarily to help doctors ascertain what stage the cancer has reached, they also have a positive impact on the patient's chances of recovery. A *lymphadenectomy*, sometimes known as lymph node dissection, involves removing some or all of the lymph nodes located in the tumour area. For example, for an ovarian tumour, the lymph nodes are removed behind the abdominal cavity adjacent to the tumour and analysed to establish the extent to which the cancer has penetrated them, which indicates whether or not the cancer has spread to other parts of the body. From a treatment perspective, removing lymph nodes from this area helps prevent the cancer from spreading via the lymphatic system.

## Prophylactic surgery

Many doctors prescribe *prophylactic surgery* as a preventative measure for people with a very high risk of contracting a particular form of cancer before it develops. By removing healthy tissue or organs that are highly likely to develop a tumour in the future, the surgery eliminates any risk of that tumour spreading and thus improves the overall health outlook of the patient.

Several surgical procedures are used to both prevent cancer and to cure it. The *salpingo-oophorectomy,* for example, is an important weapon in the fight against ovarian cancer. A *unilateral salpingo-oophorectomy* involves the removal of the ovary and fallopian tube on one side of the body—when diagnostics suggests both ovaries are at risk a *bilateral salpingo-oophorectomy* is carried out to remove both ovaries and fallopian tubes. These procedures are becoming more common as it is now apparent that more ovarian cancers originally form in the fallopian tubes, rather than the ovaries themselves, than was previously thought.

As research into how and why cancer develops—particularly the field of *cancer genomics,* which is discussed later in Chapter 8—our ability to predict who is at risk of developing which cancers, and when, improves. This in turn means prophylactic surgery is likely to become more widespread in the future. In the case of women who discover they have a high risk of developing ovarian cancer, a *bilateral salpingo-oophorectomy* is a viable option that an increasing number of women are taking up in an attempt to prevent the disease from developing.

## Curative surgery

If the staging of a tumour suggests it has not spread from its original site, there is a chance the patient can be cured by removing it. Surgeons will usually take out a small amount of healthy tissue around the tumour, known as a *margin*, to try and capture microscopic cancer cells at the tumour's extremities.

Sometimes curative surgery will also involve the removal of lymph nodes. This happens in the case of tumours located very close to lymph nodes, or those that are known not to have metastasised to another area of the body but may have spread to the nearest lymph nodes.

Curative surgery will usually be followed by a course of chemotherapy and/or radiotherapy, designed to kill off any cancerous cells that have spread beyond the confines of the tumour and the scope of the surgery.

## Cytoreductive surgery

Any tumour that is not diagnosed at an early stage in its development is likely to have spread beyond the point where it can all be safely removed surgically without causing too much damage to the body. Even small, early-stage tumours cannot always be fully removed if they are very close to major organs.

In these circumstances *cytoreductive*, or 'debulking', surgery can be performed. The aim of this process is to remove as much of the tumour as possible so other forms of treatment such as radiotherapy and chemotherapy—and, increasingly, immunotherapy and targeted therapies—are left with a smaller tumour to deal with.

## Reconstructive surgery

Surgical procedures to treat cancer can result in removal of tissue that impacts on quality of life and normal function of affected parts of the body. *Reconstructive surgery* can rectify this and is appropriate after some operations for a number of different cancers. The most widely used form of this type of surgery is breast reconstruction after a mastectomy, but it's also common for patients who have had operations to remove tumours from the head and neck and to treat skin cancers.

◆ **Microvascular surgery** is the preferred form of reconstructive surgery, and is carried out when it is possible to use tissue from elsewhere in the patient's own body. It usually involves muscle taken either from the abdominal area or from the skin on the forearm or thigh. Blood vessels are also transplanted from the donor area and connected, with the aid of a microscope, to existing blood vessels in the treatment area.

◆ **Anaplastology** is the form of reconstructive surgery required if the patient does not have suitable tissue of their own to transplant, and involves artificial implants or prostheses. Anaplastologists mould replacement body parts such as fingers, noses and teeth to replace those removed or damaged by surgery or radiation treatment.

## *Palliative surgery*

Over one-third of all cancer patients undergoing active treatment—and up to 90% of people with advanced stage cancer—experience pain. This is caused by the disease itself, such as a growing tumour causing a build-up of pressure inside the body. Pain can also be a by-product of the cancer; for example, enforced periods of inactivity can cause muscular problems. And treatment can cause pain through the high levels of radiation or doses of chemotherapy required to fight the cancer.

*Palliative surgery* is carried out to ease the pain a patient is experiencing and to reduce the symptoms their cancer brings on. This type of surgery does not cure the cancer, but it does improve quality of life. In some cases palliative surgery can increase a patient's life expectancy—although it doesn't cure the cancer, it can delay and/or prevent the potentially fatal complications that cancer can bring on.

In the case of pancreatic cancer, the bile duct may become blocked. This can result in jaundice, gallstones and a build-up of toxins in the blood. Inserting a small metal tube (a *stent*) inside the bile duct makes the patient more comfortable, as well as helping them to avoid developing these conditions.

Cancers that metastasise into the bones and cancers of the bone marrow, such as myeloma, weaken them and make them liable to easily fracture or break. A narrow titanium rod implanted through a major bone such as the femur strengthens it and gives the patient added mobility.

## TECHNOLOGY IN OPERATION

The technological advancements since the beginning of the new millennium have led to a level of precision unimaginable to surgeons even in the second half of the 20th century. Developments in fibre optics, laser technology and robotics have produced a raft of techniques that have maintained surgery's role as a pillar in the fight against cancer. So, what techniques do surgeons have at their disposal today?

## Endoscopic/laparoscopic surgery

An *endoscope* is a very thin tube containing optical fibres, which allows doctors a clear image of the inside of the body without having to open the patient up. The endoscope is inserted through one of the body's natural openings or a tiny incision, depending on the location of the tumour. It gives the surgeon a precise picture of what needs to be removed, and this is done using delicate surgical instruments that reach the target area through further tiny incisions.

Also known as *keyhole surgery*, endoscopic procedures have a number of advantages over standard open surgery: less anaesthesia, as many endoscopic procedures can be done under local, rather than general, anaesthetic; less blood loss; less pain, because of smaller scars than open surgery; a shorter hospital stay; and a quicker recovery.

As with the excisional biopsies we have discussed earlier in this chapter, different endoscopic surgical procedures depend on the location of the cancer in the body:

◆ **Video-assisted thoracoscopic surgery** enables doctors to examine the chest cavity and area around the lungs. They make two or three tiny incisions in the skin around the ribcage: through one they insert a *thoracoscope*, a thin tube with a camera in the end, to guide the procedure; through the others they use small surgical instruments to extract tissue samples for laboratory evaluation.

◆ **Endoscopic mucosal resection** is a procedure that removes tissue from anywhere in the digestive system, from the oesophagus through the stomach and down to the colon. The camera-tipped tube can be deployed to take a small sample of questionable material for diagnosis, as well as the more common purpose of surgically removing previously identified tumours.

◆ **Endoscopic tumour ablation** is employed when cancer cells have developed in the lining of the oesophagus, and cannot therefore be removed. The process uses heat, delivered by either tiny electrodes or a laser, to kill those cancerous cells. If the cancer is advanced the ablation may not kill off the cancer permanently, but the procedure can be repeated every few months as it improves the patient's quality of life by making swallowing easier.

◆ **Laparoscopic colectomy** is a minimally invasive surgical technique to treat colon cancer. A microscopic camera and surgical instruments are passed through a few tiny incisions in the abdomen and, using the image the camera transmits, surgeons carefully separate and remove the colon through a further incision. The length of colon affected by the tumour is then removed in the operating theatre before the remaining healthy colon is returned to the abdomen and reattached to the neighbouring parts of the digestive tract.

◆ **Transurethral resection** allows doctors to both diagnose and treat cancer in the bladder and the prostate. An endoscope is passed through the urethra and is used to either remove a sample of tissue for biopsy or, if cancer has already been diagnosed and is in its early stages, destroy the tumour with electric current.

## *Laser surgery*

The use of lasers instead of standard surgical instruments reduces the impact of surgery on tissue around that being operated on, and also reduces the amount of bleeding. This form of surgery also results in a significantly lower risk of infection after surgery, as it involves less contact between instruments and body tissue. Laser surgery can be carried out as a day patient—and increasingly nowadays as an outpatient—procedure, and has only minimal side effects.

Lasers deliver a high-intensity light beam that is capable of cutting through tissue—so it can be used in place of a scalpel—and also destroying cells. It is particularly effective in cytoreductive surgery, where the laser beam is used to reduce the size of tumours so they can be removed or treated with radiotherapy or chemotherapy.

Laser surgery is most commonly used to treat cancers on the surface of the skin or on the lining of internal organs. As well as shrinking established tumours in these areas, this form of treatment is capable of destroying pre-cancerous growths before they develop into fully-grown tumours.

*Photodynamic therapy* (PDT) is a tool in the treatment of basal cell carcinoma and squamous cell carcinoma in situ (Bowen's disease). The therapy involves applying a cream that makes the cells of these cancers sensitive to light, and leaving it for a few hours to allow the cream to infiltrate the cells. A laser is then directed at the area, killing those cells in less than 10 minutes of treatment and resulting in only a slight irritation that can be alleviated with a damp bandage. The process is usually repeated after a week, followed by a diagnostic procedure soon afterwards to check if all the cancerous cells have been expunged.

The initial drawback of laser surgery was that, in focusing on a very small target area and not penetrating deep into tissue, its effects were often not long-lasting and treatment had to be repeated. The carbon dioxide and argon lasers that pioneered this form of treatment do not penetrate far into the body and are, therefore, predominantly used for skin and eye conditions. However, the development of *neodymium lasers* has greatly increased the number of cancers that can be treated with laser surgery. Able to go deeper into tissue than other types of lasers, neodymium lasers are channelled through endoscopes to attack cancer cells in hard-to-reach parts of the body such as the colon and the oesophagus. The neodymium laser also facilitates rapid blood clotting, reducing the risk of internal bleeding during treatment.

### Electrosurgery

Electrosurgery is an effective tool in the treatment of small skin cancers that are diagnosed early, before they spread. The tumour is scraped off the skin's surface using a spoon-like instrument called a *curette*—a process called *curettage*. The area is then treated with heat generated by an electric current passing down a needle to burn off any remaining cancer cells and cauterise the area to prevent bleeding.

One form of electrosurgery is called LEEP—*loop electrosurgical excision procedure*. If a scan shows abnormal tissue in the cervix, for example, LEEP uses a wire loop rather than a needle for diagnosis. The loop, heated by an electrical current, cuts away the questionable tissue, which can then be tested in the laboratory to establish whether or not cervical cancer is causing the tissue abnormality.

Recovery times from electrosurgery are quicker than from more traditional forms of surgery, and bleeding is also reduced.

## Cryosurgery

Cryosurgery uses extreme cold, rather than the heat employed by laser surgery and electrosurgery, to destroy cancer cells. When used to treat external tumours such as skin cancers, it involves the application of liquid nitrogen onto the affected area. In the case of internal tumours liquid nitrogen or argon gas is delivered via a small probe called a *cryoprobe*.

Cryosurgery is used in the treatment of internal tumours when they are diagnosed early, while they are still small and have not spread. Most commonly it has been used for some bone cancers and cervical cancer, but it is also now being employed to treat early-stage prostate cancer. Doctors use ultrasound or MRI to guide the cryoprobe so healthy tissue around the tumour is not also frozen and therefore damaged.

## Robotic surgery

Robotic development in the operating theatre has significantly improved precision operations on some forms of cancer, thus reducing the impact on patients. Robotic surgery has taken the concept of *microsurgery*—operations employing a microscope to give the surgeon a clearer picture of what they are doing—to a new level, with surgical instruments deployed on remotely-controlled antennae rather than in the hands of a surgeon. All robotic surgery is *minimally invasive*, meaning it is carried out through two or more tiny incisions rather than one large cut.

Robotic surgery involves miniature, highly manoeuvrable surgical instruments guided by a surgeon using hand levers and foot pedals in the corner of the operating theatre. Before the start of the procedure, the patient's abdomen is inflated with carbon dioxide to give space in which the robot's surgical antennae can work.

Robotic systems scale down the movements of the surgeon's hands into microscopic movements inside the patient, with a camera on the antenna helping guide those movements. The console's foot pedal operates the camera and the three robotic arms that carry out the surgery are controlled by hand. Each arm is capable of gripping a wide range of miniature surgical instruments, making such systems very flexible and suitable for a variety of procedures.

The precision of robotic surgery often means the patient gets better results out of, and is able to recover more quickly from, their operation. In the case of prostate removal, for example, the system's accuracy reduces the likelihood of damage to surrounding nerves, which can result in the patient being rendered incontinent or impotent. It also leads to reduced incidence of *anastomotic leaks*—loss of important body fluids due to incisions in tissue during surgery. Patients whose prostate is removed by robotic surgery are able to return to normal activity sooner than is possible after other forms of prostatectomy. In terms of recovery time, for example, a standard prostatectomy usually results in a seven-day inpatient recovery— patients whose prostate is removed by robotic surgery can often return home within 24 hours.

On 16 February 2015, hospitals on four continents broadcast live robotic surgery on the internet, with viewers around the world not only able to watch the procedures but also to ask questions of the surgeons carrying them out via Twitter.

The operations were broadcast from ten hospitals around the world: four in Europe (in Sweden, the United Kingdom, Italy and Belgium);

three in the United States; two in Asia (in India and South Korea); and one in Australia.

At the time the event was deemed to be a ground-breaking exercise, illustrating the advantages and best-practice techniques of robotic surgery, and also helping to reassure friends and families of patients having such procedures by explaining exactly what they involve and how precise robotic surgery is. Since then, the use of robotics in the treatment of cancer has gone from being revolutionary to mainstream—by January 2019 robots had been involved in over a million surgical procedures globally—and the number of cancers they treat are growing rapidly.

In October 2018 a British man required an operation to remove all the organs in his pelvic area—including the bladder, rectum and prostate—after courses of radiotherapy and chemotherapy failed to prevent the spread of a rectal cancer. For an operation that had previously involved an incision from the chest to the pelvis and a three-week recovery in hospital, the adoption of robotic surgery for the first time in such a procedure meant just two small incisions—in his pelvis and abdomen—and being back at home within 10 days of the operation.

Robotic surgery can now be used to treat colorectal, head and neck, lung, and urological cancers. In the last couple of years robots have been used in the treatment of oesophageal cancers for the first time, and there are now three different robotic procedures used for treating thyroid cancer—when the February 2015 operation was broadcast there were none available in the fight against this form of cancer.

## NanoKnife® technology

Electrical current is used in NanoKnife® technology to kill the cancer tumour. The process uses MRI images and ultrasound scans to guide the surgeon to the exact location of the tumour. The NanoKnife®, which comprises a set of tiny electrode needles, sends a series of electrical pulses targeted at the pores of the tumour, opening them up permanently. Once the pores are open, the cancerous cells die and the tumour is destroyed.

This technology, also referred to as *focal irreversible electroporation* (IRE), was originally developed to treat prostate cancer. It not only allows the patient to keep their prostate, but also means significantly reduced side effects compared to a standard prostatectomy: the surgery is targeted at the tumour and has less impact on the rest of the prostate gland and surrounding tissue, so nerves related to urinary and erectile functions are less likely to be affected.

Having proved the efficacy of the technique in the treatment of prostate cancer, researchers set out to assess its potential in treating difficult-to-reach tumours in other solid organs. Today it is used in the pancreas, liver, lungs and kidneys—often treating tumours that were considered inoperable due to their location in vital organs until this technology was developed.

The procedure involves a shorter stay in hospital than usual surgery—in the case of very small tumours patients can be discharged the same day—and minimal post-operative discomfort.

## High intensity focused ultrasound

To destroy cancer tumours, high intensity focused ultrasound (HIFU) uses the process of *ablation*—heat treatment. Rather than using light waves that heat anything in their path, this procedure generates sound waves that produce a temperature of up to 90°C when they reach the target cells at the bottom of the large intestine, breaking them down and killing them. The treatment takes between one and four hours, depending on the size of the tumour. It is a minimally invasive treatment and patients can usually return home from hospital within 24 hours of admission.

As HIFU delivers a concentrated beam to a specific area, it is only suitable for the treatment of primary tumours and cannot be used for cancers that have spread. Its best results have been in the treatment of smaller tumours, so patients with larger ones can be prescribed a course of radiotherapy or hormone therapy to shrink the size of their tumour before undergoing a HIFU procedure. The full potential of this form of treatment is still being assessed in clinical trials taking place in various parts of the world. The Food and Drug Administration (FDA) licensed HIFU for ablation of prostate tissue in the US in October 2015, and the results of ongoing clinical trials will determine which other aspects of prostate cancer treatment the procedure will be approved for. Globally, it is now available as a prostate cancer treatment option to medical professionals conducting trials in over 50 countries and, as in the US, favourable clinical trial results suggest it will move beyond trials and specialist centres to become a more widespread treatment for the condition. Research is also taking place in a number of different countries into the viability of using HIFU in the treatment of cancers of the kidney, liver, bladder and pancreas.

◆ ◆ ◆

The development of anaesthesia in 1846 brought about a revolution in the battle against cancer, paving the way for the surgical removal of tumours being the mainstay in the treatment against most forms of the disease for over a century. And there has been a new revolution in cancer surgery since the turn of the 21st century, sparked by technology. The adoption of microscopic cameras, precision instruments and lasers has given surgeons the ability to be far more targeted and precise about what tissue they remove, and what they can leave behind. This, in turn, has made surgery far less invasive for patients—procedures can be completed in much shorter time and the recovery process accelerated.

While breakthroughs such as immunotherapy and cancer genomics have grabbed more of the headlines in recent years, surgeons have constantly been innovating towards improved outcomes and less adverse side effects for patients. The marriage of different treatment types—using chemotherapy or radiotherapy to reduce the size of tumours so they can be more easily excised, or using cytoreductive surgery to remove the part of a tumour that can be taken out, in order to improve the likelihood of a targeted therapy destroying the rest of the cancerous cells—is standard today, and makes surgery as relevant in the fight against cancer as it was a hundred years ago.

Chapter 4

# TURN ON THE RADIO
# RADIATION THERAPY

Today, radiation therapy—*radiotherapy*—is used in several ways: as a treatment in itself; to reduce the size of a tumour before surgery to remove it; and post-operatively, to try to prevent cancer returning once a tumour has been taken out.

In this chapter we will investigate how radiotherapy is used to:

◆ cure cancer

◆ control cancer, reducing its size and/or stopping its spread

◆ improve the effectiveness of another form of treatment, such as surgery

◆ relieve pain, control bleeding and relieve obstruction as a palliative measure.

To begin with, here's how radiotherapy helped Carla to travel again after an arduous cancer journey.

## Returning to *la dolce vita*

In the early 1970s Carla had just opened a restaurant in Melbourne's inner north when Alfonso, recently arrived from Sicily, bought the cake shop next door. Their eyes met when they turned up to work one day, and soon the wall between the two Lygon Street properties was knocked down. Carla and Alfonso consolidated both their businesses and their private lives, getting married within months of meeting.

At this time, the Lygon Street area was quickly transforming itself into the 'Little Italy' of today. Carla and Alfonso were instrumental in creating the Carlton Italian Festa, the annual street festival celebrating *la dolce vita* and all things Italian. By the early '80s it was attracting over a million visitors.

The couple's business thrived through the 1980s and '90s and their children came on board as they finished their studies. Carla and Alfonso travelled regularly, and a decade ago bought a property in Italy. They spend a few months of every year there, enjoying the Mediterranean summer and escaping the cold and blustery winters the Southern Ocean brings to Melbourne.

In 2012, the trip to Italy had to be cancelled. Carla had been trying to ignore some nagging discomfort in her stomach for a couple of months, but eventually she went to see her GP. He didn't like what he found and referred her to a specialist. What Carla thought was a minor irritation was diagnosed as cancer of the colon. Surgery removed the primary tumour, but a small amount of the cancer remained and follow-up treatment was needed. For 18 months she underwent a series of chemotherapy treatments.

Every month Carla would go into hospital and return home hooked up to a portable pump, which further restricted the small number of tasks she could now manage around the house. Various drugs were tried but her *cancer markers*—substances in the body that gauge the level of cancer present—would not come down.

Chemotherapy has played a key role in the survival and improved health of many cancer patients around the world, but none of the courses Carla received were effective for her.

To make matters worse, although she was told before chemotherapy that losing her hair was the worst thing that would happen, there were, in fact, far more painful and debilitating side effects.

Every patient reacts differently to chemotherapy, and different drugs have different side effects that usually fade once treatment has been completed. Among the more common experiences of patients receiving chemotherapy are tiredness and lack of energy, nausea and loss of appetite, and sensitive skin. But for Carla, the biggest issue was a lack of recall and an inability to concentrate. 'They don't tell you about the brain fog,' she says. 'It took over six months to regain normal brain function, and up to a year for some lost memories to return. I don't think some of them have come back, and I fear they never will.'

According to all the medical professionals involved in her treatment, Carla's tumour was particularly difficult to deal with. One of them described it as 'an atypical tumour which behaves in an atypical fashion'. In late 2013 she developed secondary bladder cancer. In January 2014 Carla's oncologist delivered the prognosis every patient dreads—she probably only had a few weeks left to live.

However, a new direction in Carla's treatment turned the tide in her favour. She embarked on a new course of *external beam radiation therapy* (EBRT), going hospital for four consecutive days one week each month for 20-minute sessions. Carla found the ongoing radiotherapy less daunting and a more positive experience than her chemotherapy. Treatment took place in a high-tech department where every step of the process and all the side effects were fully explained—a contrast to her experience with chemotherapy.

Most importantly, the radiotherapy worked. Carla's colon cancer markers are finally coming down. After surgery removed the worst of the bladder cancer, the radiotherapy made good progress in destroying the remains of it.

After the course of radiotherapy finished, she and Alfonso headed back to their beautiful house in the Italian hills.

Radiotherapy was first used to treat cancer in the late 1890s, within a few years of German physicist Wilhelm Röntgen discovering X-rays in 1895. However, its early use involved very large doses of radiation being administered for an hour or more—not only were there serious side effects, but it was quickly discovered that the radiation could be a cause of cancer as well as a cure. Because of this, radiotherapy was used as a *palliative measure*—to alleviate the symptoms of cancer rather than to cure it—until the middle of the 20th century.

Advances in radiation technology married to advances in computing in the second half of the 20th century meant safer and more effective radiotherapy. More targeted radiotherapy was developed, delivering a strong dose of radiation to the cancerous cells while avoiding damage to nearby healthy tissue.

## EXTERNAL RADIOTHERAPY

New methods of delivering radiotherapy make it far more targeted than was previously possible, increasing its effectiveness and reducing its side effects. A number of specialised forms of external radiotherapy are tailored to deal with different cancers.

### External beam radiation therapy

The form of radiotherapy treatment Carla received is EBRT. This is delivered using an advanced X-ray machine—a linear accelerator—that targets the cancer tumour itself with a highly focused beam of radiation. Each EBRT session only lasts a few minutes, with the frequency and number of treatments varying according to severity of symptoms. EBRT can be used as a stand-alone treatment. It is also often deployed to try and shrink a tumour prior to surgery, or to remove any vestiges of cancer and prevent it from returning after surgery. It may be used in conjunction with a course of chemotherapy to enhance the effect of the drugs.

### Three-dimensional conformal radiation therapy

Another form of EBRT is *three-dimensional conformal radiation therapy* (3DCRT), which sees beams directed in such a way that they match the shape and size of the cancerous tumour. As 3DCRT results in radiation more often hitting the tumour itself and less of the surrounding tissue, a higher dosage of radiation can be safely used— this increases the effectiveness of the treatment. 3DCRT has produced particularly good results in treatment of cancers of the head and neck, lung, liver and prostate.

## Intensity modulated radiation therapy

An advanced form of EBRT is *intensity modulated radiation therapy* (IMRT). Software programs control the intensity of individual beams, so different amounts of radiation are delivered to various parts of the targeted treatment area, enabling beams to be extensively shaped. IMRT can deliver radiation in beams from many different directions, spreading the dose out across the target area and therefore reducing the levels of radiation received by healthy cells it passes through. This form of radiotherapy is most useful in the treatment of the same cancers as 3DCRT.

## Hypofractionated radiation

Used in the treatment of patients with early breast or prostate cancer, *hypofractionated radiation* treatments involve patients receiving a larger dose of radiation in fewer sessions of treatment than traditional post-operative radiotherapy regimes. This reduces the total number of weeks a patient has to receive radiotherapy, usually from seven weeks down to between three and five. Many patients who have received hypofractionated radiation treatment show lower levels of toxicity and fewer signs of fatigue that those that result from the standard seven-week, lower-dose regimes.

For early-stage breast cancer patients, the treatment is often completed with one or two even larger doses of radiation aimed at the tissue surrounding the area where the tumour was first detected and, therefore, where the cancer would be most likely to recur. This is known as a *tumour bed boost*. Hypofractionated radiation is usually used by doctors as the final course of post-operative treatment for patients who do not require additional chemotherapy after their surgery.

## Proton beam therapy

This treatment works in a similar way to 3DCRT but uses *proton beams* rather than X-rays. Proton beams collect energy as they move through the body, releasing that accumulated energy once they hit the tumour. Proton beams are able to deliver a very high dose of radiation to the tumour with minimal impact on the surrounding tissue.

Because this form of treatment reduces the risk of damage to tissue adjoining the target area, it is particularly effective for tumours in the vicinity of very sensitive nerves. Proton beam radiation therapy is used most often to treat cancers of the eye, the head and the neck. It is also the most effective tool against *chordoma*, a rare form of cancer of the nervous system that usually develops at the base of the skull or in the lower back.

Because of its lower impact on the area around the tumour, proton beam therapy is being used more and more in the treatment of children. Their healthy tissue is more sensitive than adults because it is still developing, and therefore more susceptible to long-term damage from radiation.

## Electron beam therapy

Electron beams cannot pass through much body tissue, but are very effective in the treatment of skin cancer. In the early stages of skin cancer, when only a few small spots on the body require treatment, *electron beam therapy* (EBT) focuses electron beams on those spots— this is called *spot treatment*. In the case of some rare skin cancers the machine dispensing the electron beams will rotate around the body to treat the entire skin surface in a process known as *total skin electron beam therapy* (TSEBT).

## Image-guided radiation therapy

Frequent imaging of the target area during treatment enables increased accuracy as doctors continually redirect radiation beams. This method, *image-guided radiation therapy* (IGRT), is most effective when the cancer is in an area of the body that is constantly moving, including expanding and contracting, such as the lungs. It is also used when the tumour is close to vital organs such as the heart, to ensure beams are directed away from them and they do not receive any radiation.

In some cancers a tumour may be in a different position each time a patient comes in for treatment. For example, the position of the prostate gland in the body at any given time depends on how full the bladder is.

*Four-dimensional radiotherapy* (4D-RT) employs the three-dimensional (3-D) scanning used in IGRT to allow doctors to control where beams are being directed, and adds the fourth dimension of time to predict where the tumour will move throughout the treatment.

## TomoTherapy®

This is a form of radiation treatment that combines IMRT and CT scanning. TomoTherapy® is especially effective for tumours in hard-to-get-at parts of the body, or those that are sitting right next to vital organs.

A scan prior to the treatment generates 3-D images that are fed into software, creating a 'map' defining the contours of each tumour. From this information doctors can compute the level of radiation the tumour should receive. The treatment is then delivered in a spiral pattern, rotating around the patient so the tumour is attacked from all angles.

The whole process takes only 20 minutes or so, and as the treatment is painless—the experience is similar to that of having an X-ray or a scan—it can be administered daily if required.

TomoTherapy® is now used to treat cancers of the prostate, breast, lung, brain, and other tumours in the head and neck.

## Volumetric modulated arc therapy

Sweeping single or multiple radiation beams around the patient— *volumetric modulated arc therapy* (VMAT)—reduces the time radiation needs to be administered to be effective by much as 75%. Like IGRT, this method involves regular 3-D images being generated during treatment so dosages can be controlled and tumour locations monitored as they receive radiation.

VMAT has become—like TomoTherapy®—another important weapon in the battle against tumours that have wrapped themselves around vital organs or very sensitive parts of the body. Such tumours were unable to be treated with radiotherapy until these technologies were developed. This is due to the rotating beams and the angles that VMAT allows doctors to attack tumours from.

When it first came into widespread use a decade or so ago, VMAT was used most commonly in the treatment of liver, pancreatic and prostate cancers. Today, however, its scope has increased significantly, with the therapy also used in the treatment of tumours in the head, neck, breast and central nervous system.

### Stereotactic surgery

Despite its name, *stereotactic surgery* (SRT) is not a surgical procedure but a form of radiation treatment. A large number of individual beams focus on one target area, so it tends to be used for smaller tumours than other forms of radiotherapy, but delivers a higher dose of radiation to them.

SRT is used mainly in the treatment of brain tumours, when a specific area is targeted and nearby tissue must not receive any radiation. It is also used for spinal-cord tumours, where similar conditions exist—a small tumour surrounded by delicate tissue. Occasionally small, well-defined tumours elsewhere in the body in particularly sensitive areas are treated in the same way, with multiple beams focusing on the same spot. In these situations the treatment is called *stereotactic body radiotherapy* (SBRT) or *stereotactic ablative radiotherapy* (SABR).

### CyberKnife®

A new development in SRT is CyberKnife®. The patient is scanned before treatment, and a 3-D model of their inside made. Doctors can then plan the path of each of the hundreds of individual beams that converge on the target area of the treatment. This puts CyberKnife® among the most accurate vehicles delivering radiotherapy—in standard forms of the treatment, the area one centimetre from the heart of the beam receives 60% of the radiation at the centre; that ratio is reduced to 10% using CyberKnife®.

The technology incorporates finely-tuned sensors that can track movements within the body, such as a respiring lung. The sensors transmit this information to the source of the radiotherapy beams so they oscillate and are continuously delivered to the target area and not the surrounding tissue.

The accuracy and effectiveness of CyberKnife® means that fewer incidents of treatment in a shorter period of time are required than for more traditional forms of radiotherapy. The usual course is three 45-minute treatments administered once a week.

## Prophylactic cranial irradiation

Another form of external radiotherapy is *prophylactic cranial irradiation* (PCI), which delivers high-energy X-rays to the whole brain to destroy any microscopic cancer cells that have spread to it.

Doctors often recommend PCI once a lung cancer patient has been successfully treated and is in remission. Lung cancer patients who have gone into remission have a 60% chance of the disease recurring in the brain after two years.

When lung cancer metastasises, one of the places it most often spreads to is the brain. No form of cancer treatment guarantees that every malignant cell is destroyed, and because symptoms can take years to present, the cancer may have spread undetected before it is treated in its primary location.

The results of a trial involving more than 700 patients with small cell lung cancer (SCLC)—some with the disease at an early stage and others advanced—were reported in June 2020. Participants in the trial with early-stage SCLC who received PCI had a 21% better survival rate than those who didn't have the treatment, and those with an advanced stage of the disease who had the PCI therapy had a 14% better survival rate than those who didn't.

### Microbeam radiation therapy

An extremely advanced form of radiotherapy is *microbeam radiation therapy* (MRT). As it is yet to be fully trialled it isn't, therefore, available to patients at time of writing. Nevertheless, MRT is causing waves in the scientific community and the results of research into the therapy conducted to date suggest it could become a major weapon in the battle against cancer within the next decade.

MRT involves very-high-dose X-rays combined with micron-sized beams that provide an unprecedented level of precision in terms of the area being targeted. By being able to strike a much smaller area than has previously been possible, doctors will be able to administer far higher doses of radiation. Pre-clinical evidence from MRT tests reveals that the technology behind it leads to a significant reduction in the damage to normal tissue.

A study at Melbourne's Australian Nuclear Science and Technology Organisation Synchrotron radiation facility in late 2018 showed that MRT could safely deliver radiation doses up to 20 times higher than existing forms of radiotherapy. The research—a combined exercise led by the Royal Women's Hospital, RMIT University and University of Melbourne—is expected to lead to authorities giving the green light to a human trial of MRT in Australia. The head of the Synchrotron, Professor Andrew Peele, said that the research 'has the potential to improve cancer treatment and make the experience more comfortable and effective for patients', and the team behind the research predicted that MRT would be the first step on a path that will ultimately lead to cancer patients needing just a single radiotherapy treatment.

## INTERNAL RADIOTHERAPY

Internal radiotherapy delivers a high-intensity dose of radiation directly to the area around the tumour. It involves either the physical implant of a radioactive source—*brachytherapy*—or delivery of a radioactive liquid into the body via swallowing a capsule or an injection.

The term *brachytherapy* means short-distance therapy. Unlike external radiotherapy beams that pass through the body, an internal implant places the radioactive source right next to the target area. Implants can be either permanent or temporary:

**Permanent brachytherapy**: a pellet or seed, approximately the size of a grain of rice, is implanted into the tumour itself. It releases radioactivity into the tissue until it runs out, at which point the tiny and harmless seed or pellet remains embedded.

**Temporary brachytherapy**: a needle or catheter is implanted into the tumour. Doctors place a radioactive source inside the needle or catheter for a set period of time, then take it out again. Once the course of treatment is complete, the radioactive source and its container are removed.

The permanent method releases a continuous dose of radioactivity over a long period of time, whereas temporary brachytherapy allows doctors to control and vary the dose, and how long it is released into the body for. The advantage of the direct delivery of the radioactive source into the tumour is the high dose that can be administered, as there is a rapid fall-off in the dose that reaches adjoining tissue. Generally 90% of the dose is concentrated within one centimetre of the source.

Brachytherapy alone is capable of curing some cancers that are diagnosed early, when the tumour is still in its primary location and has not started to spread. It is still used in more entrenched cancers that have grown and spread, but in these cases it is usually one of a combination of treatment types, which often include surgery. In these circumstances it is effective in reducing the size of the tumour and preventing it from causing obstructions to airways or the digestive-system tracts.

Brachytherapy is most commonly used to treat cervical, prostate, breast and skin cancer—all cancers in parts of the body relatively accessible for delivery of implants. There is, however, a form of brachytherapy that is used to treat lung cancer, using an ingenious device to treat this harder-to-access part of the body.

*Endobronchial therapy* delivers a dose of internal radiation to the lung cancer tumour. A catheter is placed down the throat and radioactive pellets injected into the catheter by a brachytherapy control machine called an *afterloader*. The catheter is manoeuvred so it delivers the pellets into direct contact with the tumour. Once treatment is complete, which is usually five to 10 minutes depending on the size of the tumour, the afterloader withdraws the pellets.

## Selective internal radiotherapy

Specifically to treat liver cancer, *selective internal radiotherapy treatment* (SIRT) involves the use of minute pellets, or microspheres. They are placed inside a catheter that is then inserted into the hepatic artery, which supplies the liver with blood from the heart. The microspheres deliver a high dose of radiation that interferes with the supply of fresh blood to the cancerous tumour, causing it to shrink. This process is called *radioembolisation*.

The main difference between SIRT and other forms of internal radiotherapy is its effectiveness on its own in the treatment of advanced secondary tumours. Many liver cancers have metastasised from primary tumours elsewhere in the body, most commonly the breast and lung. SIRT is proving to be effective against liver tumours that cannot be removed surgically and that are resistant to chemotherapy. The liver is extremely sensitive to radiation, so external radiotherapy techniques cannot be used in these cases—the microspheres travel through the blood directly into the tumour and have less of an impact on the surrounding liver tissue.

## Partial breast irradiation

One form of internal radiotherapy suitable for breast cancer patients who have had a *lumpectomy*—removal of a tumour that has not yet metastasised from the breast—is partial breast irradiation. This is administered twice a day for a week and specifically targets the area of the breast from which the lump has been removed. The preparation for partial breast irradiation is done during, or soon after, the lump-removal surgery. A tiny device is implanted in the place from which the lump is removed. The treatment involves a radioactive seed being placed in the device during treatments, and removed between them. The device is removed once the course of radiotherapy is complete.

### *Radioisotope therapy*

*Radioisotopes* are radioactive sources delivered in liquid form, delivered either orally as a drink or capsule or intravenously through an injection. The radioactive element is then delivered to the cancerous tissue by the bloodstream.

The most commonly used radioisotope therapy is a radioactive iodine that is used in the treatment of thyroid cancer. A similar compound has also been found to be effective against *neuroblastoma*— a cancer that usually occurs in infants and young children and that makes up almost 10% of all paediatric cancer cases—and *lymphoma,* a blood cancer that affects the lymphatic system. Radioisotopes are also regularly used to treat secondary bone cancers.

## RADIOSENSITISERS

Radiotherapy works by damaging the DNA of malignant cells, the DNA being the basic building blocks of life found in the nucleus of cells. All cells in the body, both healthy and cancerous, have a highly efficient repair process that continually protects and renews DNA as it comes into constant contact with potentially harmful chemicals moving around the body. *Radiosensitisers* interfere with the DNA repair process, increasing the chances that radiotherapy will kill the cancerous cells.

Initially the development of radiosensitisers focused on oxygen diffusion-enhancing compounds. Tumours grow at such a rate that they operate in an environment starved of oxygen, known as *hypoxia*, and scientists found this state significantly contributed to their ability to resist radiotherapy. The fundamental aim of radiosensitisers is to combat this resistance by increasing oxygen levels in cancerous cells.

Today researchers are looking to develop new compounds that mimic the impact of oxygen but are more efficient, as oxygen itself is rapidly consumed by cells. They are looking for *cytotoxins*—chemical agents that have a toxic effect—that act as a catalyst with radiation doses to increase lethal damage in tumour cells.

Scientists are also working to develop *radioprotectors*, compounds that protect healthy tissue from the harmful effects of radiation. In theory, radioprotectors will enable higher doses of radiation than can currently be used safely, thereby increasing the effectiveness of the treatment.

◆ ◆ ◆

Radiotherapy has come a long way since its early days. A high dose of radiation no longer blitzes the area of the body where a tumour is located, affecting not just the cancer but the tissue surrounding it and the tissue it passes through to reach it.

Technology has enabled radiographers to target cancer cells more precisely, and to treat patients with radioactive elements that are far less harmful than the primitive ones used originally.

Advances in imaging allow them to identify smaller tumours that went undetected in the past, and also enable them to look at the areas as they are treating them and adjust the direction and intensity of the treatment as it progresses.

Combining radiotherapy with surgery, chemotherapy and immunotherapy is a major component of the integrated approach to cancer treatment that gives better outcomes than when single treatment types are employed at any one time.

Ongoing research to hone existing techniques and to develop new forms of radiotherapy—and to optimise its use in combination with other forms of treatment—will ensure it remains one of the cornerstones of the fight against cancer in the years to come.

## Chapter 5

# HITTING THE TARGET CHEMOTHERAPY

The general term *chemotherapy* means drugs that kill cells. Its basic premise is to attack the DNA in cancerous cells so they stop their ongoing growth and division, in effect causing them to 'commit suicide'. A better understanding of the way chemotherapy impacts on cells and our DNA means some of the new chemotherapy drugs cross over into personalised medicine and immunotherapy. This new generation of drugs is known as *targeted therapies*.

In this chapter we will delve into:

◆ the breakthrough that launched chemotherapy

◆ the key role chemotherapy plays in the treatment of the 'big five' cancers

◆ the way targeted therapies reduce side effects for the patient.

First, here's Jeremy's story of how chemotherapy gave him a second chance.

## Eight times lucky

Four years ago Jeremy started to suffer from mild back pain. He thought this was ironic—he had recently started exercising at the gym in an attempt to look after his health after a decade of inactivity.

'I played football and cricket at school, and got into squash when I was at university,' he says. 'I carried on with that through my twenties, but developed a knee problem and had to give it away when I was 32.'

Jeremy's career really took off around this time—he worked long hours and spent the time he did have away from the office socialising. 'Initially I really missed the squash, but didn't replace it with anything and pretty quickly I was living a full life, but one without any worthwhile exercise.' It was Jeremy's doctor who persuaded him, during a consultation about some inoculations for an overseas holiday, that getting back into some regular exercise would be very good for his long-term wellbeing.

To begin with, Jeremy changed his routine in the gym so he didn't exacerbate the back problem, hoping that whatever was causing the pain would right itself. When that didn't happen he went to the physio, but they were unable to identify the problem. He started to feel generally unwell and a work colleague told him that he 'looked a funny colour'. The following morning Jeremy himself noticed his eyes looked yellow in the mirror, and he made an appointment to see his GP.

The doctor told Jeremy he had jaundice, but that a comprehensive round of tests would be required to identify the underlying condition that had brought it about. After a few weeks, when nothing was confirmed but a lot of things ruled out, Jeremy started to lose his appetite and feel progressively worse. A CT scan was arranged.

The results of the scan were a double blow for Jeremy. Not only did he have pancreatic cancer, but the tumour was too big to be operated on by the time it had been discovered. Jeremy's oncologist prescribed a regime of chemotherapy consisting of a combination of three drugs, with the aim of reducing the tumour to a size that would enable surgery to remove it.

The chemotherapy was administered in three-week cycles. The first two weeks of each cycle involved Jeremy going into hospital to receive intravenous doses of two of the drugs, while he took the third in tablet form. Although Jeremy was only actually in hospital for half a day on the first visit of each cycle, and just a few hours a week later for the second, it took him days to get over each visit. The evening after treatment wasn't too bad, but then Jeremy would 'really hit the wall' and have a couple of days when he felt exhausted and didn't leave the house, especially in the first couple of treatment cycles.

Throughout the eight months he received chemotherapy Jeremy constantly had mild cold-like symptoms, and he says he couldn't taste very much although he retained his sense of smell. This made it even harder to keep eating, bearing in mind his lack of appetite, but he knew he had to keep his strength up and told himself that eating was supplementing his treatment. He lost about 20 kilos but was strong enough to get himself around, seeing friends from time to time, occasionally going into the office—mostly working from home— and regularly getting some fresh air.

Jeremy believes that carrying on doing some work throughout his chemotherapy treatment helped him keep his spirits up and retain a sense of perspective. 'I don't think I would have got through it if I didn't have something else to focus on,' he says. 'My boss and my colleagues were amazing, not putting any pressure on me but still emailing me for my thoughts on things and giving me first shot at some of the tasks I was doing before.

'Although I was aware the absolute priority was to try and get better, I thought I would just be consumed if that was all I thought about. I needed a sense of purpose, and challenging myself to get a little bit of work done while I was going through the chemo made me feel better about myself, which made me feel better in myself.'

Another positive was the fact that, after a couple of months, the chemotherapy was having some effect. The second scan showed that the tumour had shrunk a little, and that gave Jeremy the impetus to tolerate the side effects more easily. He says the round of hospital visits, taking his tablets, and even the days after treatment when he was exhausted became part of his routine.

After eight cycles of chemotherapy the tumour had shrunk sufficiently for Jeremy to undergo surgery. He had a pancreaticoduodenectomy—known as the Whipple procedure, named after the person who first performed it in the United States in the 1930s—to remove the head of his pancreas, his duodenum and part of his stomach that surrounded the tumour.

Jeremy is well aware that his cancer could come back in the future, and it took him a long time to recover from his surgery—the Whipple procedure is a complex one and a major operation—but he is getting on with life, and work. He is very thankful for the chemotherapy that has at least given him a chance of being cured and is making the most of what he describes as his 'second chance'.

———————

'Cancer cells are pretty messed up,' says Professor Jonathan Cebon, Head of the Cancer Immunobiology Program at the Olivia Newton-John Cancer Research Institute in Melbourne. 'Whereas a normal cell that recognises it has lots of damage will commit suicide, to avoid that damage having any ramifications for the rest of the body, a cancerous cell gets rid of the mechanism that enables it to kill itself and goes all out for survival—basically, it goes rogue.

'Because it causes itself more and more damage as it fights for survival, it loses the ability to defend itself against attacks on its DNA, which has already been damaged by chemotherapy,' Professor Cebon explains. 'That is why chemotherapy kills cancer cells and not the patient—the healthy cells are able to protect their DNA from the attack on it by the chemotherapy as they still have the sense and the ability to fix themselves; the cancer cells reach a point where they are so degraded that they cannot survive.'

## A WWII BREAKTHROUGH

A bombing raid in Italy during World War II resulted in a stockpile of nitrogen mustard, developed by both sides in the war but never used offensively, being released into the air. Autopsies on victims of this incident revealed that the compound had significantly reduced the division of cells in their lymphatic systems, and was the first hint that the use of chemicals may be able to adopted in the treatment of cancer.

As a result of the research prompted by this event, a compound of nitrogen mustard became the first chemotherapy drug. From the mid-1940s onwards chemotherapy was the main focus of cancer treatment, on the basis that if you could kill infections using drugs you should be able to kill cancers with them as well. This model has proved to only work with a limited numbers of cancers—most notably childhood leukaemias, lymphomas and germ cell tumours (such as testicular cancer)—but was not the universal cure-all it was hoped to be.

## 1960S DEVELOPMENT

In the 1960s it was discovered that platinum reacts to the bacteria in which cells live to create an environment in which the cells cannot grow and divide—and platinum derivatives have been a mainstay of many chemotherapy treatments ever since. In the early days specific drugs were used against different cancers, but years of funding and of research have resulted in the development of chemotherapy drugs and targeted therapies that are more versatile than their predecessors, with some of these drugs now proving to be effective against different cancers.

When Imatinib was authorised for use by the US FDA in 2001 it was specifically designed to treat a rare form of leukaemia that affects certain white blood cells, but it has since proved to be effective against multiple forms of cancers. It is now used in the treatment of gastrointestinal stromal tumours (GISTs)—cancers that start in the walls of the digestive system and spread elsewhere in the body from there—and dermatofibrosarcoma protuberans (DFSP), a rare form of cancer that forms in the middle layer of the skin (*dermis*). Researchers are now also investigating using the drug to treat pulmonary hypertension, one of the major causes of heart attacks and strokes.

Trabectedin was licensed for use by the European Medicines Evaluation Agency in 2007, and is now prescribed to patients with most of the different forms of soft tissue sarcomas. These diseases are caused by malignant tumours that develop from muscles, nerves, fat, blood vessels or the skin, and the one drug is used to treat many of the sarcomas that start in these different body tissues. The drug binds itself to the DNA of cancerous cells, preventing them from multiplying and growing. Trabectedin is also used to treat ovarian cancer patients whose disease has developed resistance to platinum-based drugs.

## A TARGETED APPROACH

A greater understanding of the fundamental biology of cells is helping doctors to influence how cancers behave, and how the body's immune system identifies and reacts to them. As we learn more about the science behind the disease, researchers are coming up with new drugs that hit the cancer cells more accurately, reducing the impact on healthy cells.

Targeted therapies fight cancer in specific ways, targeting individual proteins that affect the way cancer cells function and making them behave differently to normal, healthy cells.

A number of specialist clinics around the world are now having some success in predicting which chemotherapy treatments will work for individual patients. They conduct biopsies of small tumour samples sent to them, often from overseas, and report back to the hospital treating the patient. They recommend which specific course of chemotherapy is most appropriate for that patient, removing the 'trial and error' aspect that was an inevitable part of treatment plans for so long.

The view for many years was that the *cytotoxic* (cell-destroying) chemotherapy killed cancer cells by poisoning them. Today, however, emerging evidence proves that the drugs affect the patient's immune system, helping spark the immune system into fighting the cancer rather than killing it themselves. *Monoclonal antibody drugs* are targeted therapies that are made in the lab but which resemble proteins in the body's immune system, in effect 'rearming' the immune system by increasing its weaponry to fight the cancer.

## CHEMOTHERAPY AND THE 'BIG' CANCERS

The American Cancer Society calls cancers of the lung, breast, prostate and bowel the *big four* because of the large numbers of people who have developed them compared to other forms of the disease. These most common forms of cancer have not been significantly impacted themselves by chemotherapy. Where chemotherapy has been, and continues to be, useful against them is as an *adjuvant therapy*: giving chemotherapy as a follow-up to reduce the danger of relapse in patients considered high-risk after attempts to cure their cancer with surgery and/or radiotherapy.

In recent years great strides have been made in developing therapies to fight the big four, helping to reduce their mortality rates around the world. Globally, the mortality rate from these forms of cancer has dropped significantly in recent decades:

◆ For non-small cell lung carcinoma (NSCLC)—the most common type of lung cancer—deaths dropped by 51% among men and 26% among women between 2000 and 2020.

◆ For breast cancer, deaths fell by 40% between 1989 and 2019.

◆ For prostate cancer in the US, deaths fell by more than 50% between 1993 and 2017.

◆ For people over the age of 50 with bowel cancer, deaths fell by 32% between 2000 and 2013.

In all forms of the disease, a combination of factors brought about the reduction—in prostate cancer, for example, advances in robotic surgical techniques have played a large part—but more targeted therapies used in conjunction with other treatment have played an equally important role.

### If the cap fits...

One of the most troubling side effects of some chemotherapy or radiotherapy drugs may be *chemotherapy-induced alopecia*—hair loss.

Hair may be lost from anywhere on the body—from the scalp, eyebrows and lashes and face to the chest, underarms and pubic area. The amount of hair loss depends on the type of drug, dose and timing of treatment cycles. This is because any treatment that acts on rapidly dividing cancer cells will also affect rapidly dividing hair follicles.

Scalp cooling (scalp hypothermia) is intended to prevent or slow hair loss from the scalp. It works by narrowing the blood vessels and thus reducing the amount of drug reaching the scalp. Cold caps and other scalp-cooling systems are applied before, during and following treatment.

Not everyone is suited to scalp cooling as it can cause headaches and faintness or nausea, extend treatment time by hours and chill the body too much. Some people may still experience hair thinning, or partial or total hair loss.

The success rate is not well established, with so many different drugs and other variables. However, Peter MacCallum Cancer Centre quotes some evidence that scalp cooling can lower the risk of significant hair loss by 43%, leaving people feeling that they had enough remaining hair so they did not need to use a wig or hair covering.

Everyone's situation is different—health professionals are the best people to advise.

## TARGETED THERAPIES

Many of the breakthroughs in the development of targeted therapies have resulted from research into the fight against the big four cancers, as you'll see on the next pages. However, as these therapies are further developed, they often prove to be effective against multiple forms of cancer.

### Angiogenesis inhibitors (lung and bowel cancer)

*Angiogenesis* is the process by which new blood vessels are formed. It is a key step in the development and growth of cancer tumours, and the way they spread from their primary position to other parts of the body.

*Angiogenesis inhibitors* work in one of three ways:

◆ blocking the vital protein—called *vascular endothelial growth factor* (VEGF)—that is required for blood vessels to grow

◆ preventing VEGF from transmitting its growth command signal to cells in the blood vessel

◆ stopping signals transmitted between neighbouring cells that tell each other to grow.

Angiogenesis inhibitors are unable to cure cancers by themselves, so they do not destroy tumours, but trial results show they will be effective in slowing the growth and limiting the spread of cancers.

Initially a couple of angiogenesis inhibitors were approved by the FDA for the treatment of colorectal and kidney cancers. That success led to a number of clinical trials looking at the potential of this type of compound as a treatment for other cancers, and in recent years the agency has approved more than a dozen angiogenesis inhibitors to treat various different cancers.

### Anti-epidermal growth factor receptor therapies (lung, breast and bowel cancer)

*Epidermal growth factor receptors* (EGFRs) are proteins that help cells grow and divide. This process of growth and division happens at a rapid, uncontrolled rate in cancerous cells, and in some lung cancer cells an excess of EGFRs exacerbates this problem. The drugs used to block the signal from the EGFRs that tell the cells to grow and divide are particularly effective in people who have a specific mutation in the EGFR gene—a mutation that is more common in women and non-smokers—as the mutation is the main driver in the development of cancer for those people who have it.

*Human epidermal growth factor receptor 2* (HER2) is a key protein in the growth and multiplication of cells in the breast. A mutation in the HER2 gene that makes the protein causes it to produce too much of it, a problem called *overexpression*. The excess HER2 receptors make the cells grow and multiply at an uncontrollable rate, bringing on breast cancer.

Trastuzumab is a drug that attaches itself to the surface of the breast cancer cells, blocking them and thereby preventing them from receiving further signals from the HER2 receptors to grow and multiply. Up to 20% of all cases of breast cancer are brought about by an overexpression of the HER2 gene, and two large studies completed in 2014 revealed that patients treated with a combination of chemotherapy and trastuzumab had longer life expectancy and a higher chance of getting rid of all their cancer than those who received chemotherapy alone.

A number of anti-EGFR drugs have subsequently been approved for the treatment of different cancers. For example, Cetuximab is used to treat some colorectal and head and neck cancers, in addition to metastatic lung cancer. Erlotinib was originally licensed to treat metastatic lung cancer, but the approval has subsequently also been extended for use in the treatment of pancreatic cancer as well. Afatinib has been approved in many countries around the world for metastatic lung cancer patients, and is now showing promising signs in trials for breast cancer patients with a particular gene mutation, so it may well be more widely used in the near future.

### Selective estrogen receptor modulators (breast cancer)

The most important step forward in the development of drugs to fight breast cancer in recent years has been the use of *selective estrogen receptor modulators* (SERMs). They are prescribed as a preventative measure for people who have an increased risk of breast cancer, and also as a treatment to stop the disease returning in patients who have already developed breast cancer and received treatment for it. SERMs have proved to be particularly effective in preventing *contralateral breast cancer*, stopping the disease from developing in the second breast when it has been diagnosed and treated on one side.

Estrogen (also spelled oestrogen) is a key component in the development of breast cancer, acting as the signal that tells cancerous cells to grow and multiply. SERMs attach themselves to estrogen receptors in the cells in the breast, preventing the estrogen from reaching them and passing on its signal. The term 'selective' in the description of these compounds arises because they do not behave in the same way throughout the body: they do not block estrogen from reaching cells elsewhere, and in some places do the opposite, promoting a response to the estrogen. In breast cells, however, they are highly effective and now widely used. The most common SERMs prescribed to patients are Tamoxifen and Raloxifene, and can be used before, during and after menopause.

## Aromatase inhibitors (breast cancer)

*Aromatase inhibitors* were only developed very late in the 20th century. Originally used to treat existing cancers, they are now also proving effective in reducing the risk of cancer recurring in women who have been treated for early-stage breast cancer. Although not yet approved as drugs that can be taken to prevent cancer in women who don't have cancer but are at risk of doing so, trials into their suitability for this purpose are underway. Aromatase inhibitors only work in post-menopausal women, i.e. those whose bodies are no longer producing estrogen, but they have proved highly effective in these situations and have fewer side effects than other forms of treatment.

Aromatase is an enzyme in the body that converts hormones into estrogen. The aromatase inhibitors reduce the levels of estrogen in the body by stopping this process, thus reducing the number of signals estrogen gives to cancerous cells to grow and multiply. Aromatase inhibitors have proved to be the most effective type of drug developed to date in the treatment of advanced cases of breast cancer. And when they are prescribed after SERMs have been used for a number of years, they reduce the likelihood of a patient's breast cancer coming back.

### Bisphosphonates (breast and prostate cancer)

When breast, lung or prostate cancers metastasise, the bones are one of the most common parts of the body they spread to. This causes weakness and the increased likelihood of fractures. Breakdown of bones also releases higher than usual levels of calcium into the bloodstream, causing nausea and drowsiness.

Bisphosphonates are a class of drug already used in the treatment of a number of conditions involving fragile bones, such osteoporosis, and they are now proving to be effective in the treatment of *myeloma*—a blood cancer that develops in bone marrow—and cancers that have spread to the bones from other parts of the body.

One of the most regularly used bisphosphonates is zoledronic acid, and scientists believe it may have additional uses in breast cancer treatment: studies in the US suggest it helps some hormone therapies and chemotherapy drugs to be more effective when used in conjunction with them. Research into this class of compounds continues, with early trials resulting in a reduction in the relative risk of breast cancer recurrence of almost 15%.

### Anti ADT-resistant drugs (prostate cancer)

The *androgen receptor* is the key element in the growth and development of prostate cancer. *Androgen deprivation therapy* (ADT) has been a cornerstone in treatment of the condition for many years, but tumours can develop resistance to this form of hormone therapy. Researchers have learned that tumours counter ADT over time by increasing the number of androgen receptors they produce, overwhelming the therapy.

The FDA has approved three drugs in recent years that the American Cancer Society describes as 'newer anti-androgens', which have proved to be effective in the treatment of tumours that have built up resistance to ADT. Two of these drugs are sufficiently potent to reduce PSA levels in patients with advanced prostate cancers.

# OVERCOMING DRUG-RESISTANT CELLS

The biggest challenge facing chemotherapy is the resistance that cancer cells develop to it. A number of recent developments could pave the way for developing drugs to target cells that do not respond to existing chemotherapy.

## Identifying proteins

One of the approaches to overcoming the problem is to identify the specific proteins in cancer cells that make them resistant to chemotherapy, then to create targeted therapies to nullify those proteins. Research conducted in the UK in 2014 focused on a protein called BID, and its role in *mitosis*—the process by which cells replicate and divide. Mitosis in healthy cells is a carefully controlled process, and any failure of cells to complete mitosis correctly can lead to the development of cancer. This work has subsequently been taken up and expanded upon by a number of different institutions, and in 2019 researchers at the Massachusetts Institute of Technology made a breakthrough: their modelling suggested that combining two existing types of drugs would be more effective than each of those drugs in isolation, without harming healthy cells as they divide in a different way to cancerous cells. That research team intends to start a clinical trial with a view to developing a drug combination to target mutations in tumours and remove their resistance to chemotherapy.

Another protein that scientists have had in their sights is one that pumps foreign substances out of cells. This protein, called P-Glycoprotein, carries out an important function in healthy cells by removing any harmful substances that try to infiltrate them. However, the protein is itself harmful for a cancer patient—it can act as a barrier to chemotherapy, removing the drug from the tumour cell before it has a chance to act. A number of therapies have been developed recently to counteract the action of P-Glycoprotein in cancer cells.

A problem can arise in cancer cells that prevents chemotherapy from reaching them in the first place. A mutation in proteins that are supposed to transport the drugs through the cell wall can mean that they do not carry out this function. Researchers are working to try and develop targeted therapies that override mutated transporter proteins and enable delivery of 100% of the prescribed dose of chemotherapy to tumours that currently have this form of resistance.

## Getting the timing right

A new area of focus in trials is the timing of exactly when chemotherapy is given to patients. The increasing knowledge about the different stages of cancer cells gives scientists the opportunity to develop therapies that target specific stages in tumour development. This means that identifying when the stages are taking place, not just what they are, is important so that the therapies can be administered at the most opportune moment.

Timing is also of extreme importance in the new era of combination treatments. Most combinations of different drugs, or drugs and therapies, are only effective in a window when the impact of one makes the cancer cells most vulnerable to the other(s). The ideal time for delivering the second treatment is not necessarily immediately after the first—in some cases the initial drug or therapy may take days to degrade the cancer cells to the point at which the second treatment will be most effective.

## Exploiting nanomedicine

Hopefully, however, in the future patients will not have to make repeat hospital visits to receive the different drugs and/or therapies. *Nanomedicine* harnesses the latest developments in *nanotechnology*—the manipulation of individual atoms and molecules—and one of its potential applications is a single method of delivery that gives the patient two different drugs, even when they need to be released into the cancer cells at separate times. The first drug is on the surface of the nanoparticle and goes to work as soon the patient receives the treatment, whereas the second is protected by a chemical that takes longer for the body to break down, delaying its release.

Alongside convenience for patients, the potential improvements in the delivery of chemotherapy nanomedicine are expected to offer another major advantage. Early research is showing that its ability to deliver therapies directly into cancer cells reduces the side effects they cause. Delivering specific doses of targeted therapies directly into tumours will have less impact on surrounding tissue and the white cell blood count than existing chemotherapy.

Chemotherapy nanomedicine is in its early stages—the multiple-therapy-delivery system has not yet progressed to human trials—but the results of initial testing are positive and it is an area of research that scientists around the world are putting a lot of time and effort into. For example, the author of a study conducted at the University of Helsinki said in 2019 that his team's research unveiled 'the potential of… nanoparticles to act as drug carriers to improve the anticancer drug efficacy'. And a joint Japanese/French initiative reported in early 2020 that its initial testing could 'open the doors to future therapeutic applications' of chemotherapy nanoscience.

◆ ◆ ◆

Chemotherapy has been the mainstay of cancer treatment for a long time. It is still an essential part of treatment for many cancers, although advances in surgical techniques, radiotherapy and immunotherapy have reduced the reliance that the medical profession places on chemotherapy.

Recent years have seen improvements in the effectiveness of the drugs themselves, and the accuracy with which chemotherapy can be targeted. In addition, we have increased the knowledge of how it can be harnessed with other forms of treatment to have a bigger impact on cancer than when used in isolation. As these enhancements in chemotherapy progress, it is likely to continue to play an important role in cancer treatment, and to do so with fewer, less harmful side effects for patients.

Chapter 6

# HELPING THE BODY FIGHT BACK
# IMMUNOTHERAPY

Until the late 20th century there were three main pillars in the treatment of cancer: surgery, radiotherapy and chemotherapy. The new millennium, however, has seen the development of therapies that empower the body to 'fight its own battle' against cancer. Immunotherapy treatment—also known as *biological therapy*—is now widely recognised as a key weapon in cancer specialists' armoury. It has come so far in a relatively short space of time as to be considered the fourth pillar in the fight against cancer.

In this chapter we explore how immunotherapy can:

◆ 'teach' the immune system to identify and attack specific cancer cells

◆ boost the immune system to learn to deal with tumours

◆ combat the process that allows cancer cells to 'disguise' themselves.

Before we look in detail at immunotherapy, we reveal how it, in the form of a stem cell transplant, enabled a teacher incapacitated by myeloma to get back on her feet again.

## Bouncing back from a fall

In December 2008, Alison slipped over while on a family holiday. It seemed like an innocuous fall but the pain was intense and her arm was broken. This had the potential to be incredibly inconvenient to a full-time teacher and a mother of five school-aged kids, but Alison was too busy to let it get in the way. The family returned home to

Melbourne, where they all pitched in to ensure the injury didn't stop them carrying on living life to the full.

Alison has always paid a great deal of attention to her health and fitness, and she cannot recall ever having to take a day off work before this incident. She was curious to know why a low-impact incident had resulted in a broken bone. Her orthopaedic surgeon took a scan and discovered what he thought was a benign cyst, which seemed to explain the cause of the weakness.

A couple of months later, however, another fall left Alison in agony once again, and this time her leg was broken. Now Alison had suffered two breaks in a short space of time, in situations where she would have expected to bounce straight back up with just a scrape or a bruise. In April 2009 extensive tests were carried out, including a biopsy of the bone marrow, which revealed that Alison was suffering from myeloma.

*Myeloma* is a cancer of the blood's plasma cells. The plasma cells, found in the bone marrow in the middle of the major bones in the body, are where all blood cells form. Myeloma differs from most other cancers in that it does not involve the growth of a tumour. Instead, it results in the build-up in the bone marrow of abnormal antibodies called *paraproteins*—abnormal proteins that do not fight infections like usual antibodies. The most debilitating symptoms of myeloma are bone pain, most commonly in the back, hips and skull; bone weakness; high levels of calcium in the blood, which can cause dizziness, weakness and kidney problems; and pressure on the spinal cord, which affects the nerves running down the spine.

The diagnosis was an enormous shock. Alison's first thoughts were how much her family relied on her, how they would cope if she were seriously incapacitated and, worst of all, the effect on her children if they lost a parent when they were so young. She resolved that she would throw everything at fighting the condition and making the best of things, driven by the combination of her positive outlook on life and determination to not leave her family in the lurch.

The most pressing need was to prevent small bumps and scrapes leading to broken bones. Alison had to stay mobile, to get to and from treatment for the myeloma and to keep contributing to family life. She had surgery to reinforce her hip and *femur*—the major bone in the upper leg linking the hip and the knee—with the insertion of titanium implants.

Having addressed the immediate threat to Alison's ability to stay on her feet and get around, the next step was to attack the cancer in the bone marrow of the limbs she had broken. The kids were surprised when Mum came home one day with tattoos, but this was no devil-may-care reaction to the diagnosis of a serious condition: the marks on Alison's skin were made by radiologists to identify exactly where the two-week course of radiotherapy that constituted the next stage of her treatment should be targeted.

At this time Alison was also offered the opportunity to take part in the clinical trial of the drug Revlimid®—early tests had indicated that it could be effective in curbing the proliferation of myeloma tumours. The trial was being conducted simultaneously in cities across North America and Europe as well as in Melbourne, with hospitals in Houston, Toronto, Toulouse and Athens among those involved.

After the radiotherapy and the Revlimid® trial, which lasted four months, a third front was opened in the fight to get rid of as much as possible of the cancer in Alison's bone marrow. She received an intensive course of inpatient chemotherapy, carried out over a weekend. These few days in hospital were the precursor to a couple of longer stays, which made up the critical part of Alison's treatment—a stem cell transplant.

To begin with, Alison underwent five days of *aphaeresis*, a form of transfusion that allows doctors to break a patient's blood down and extract certain components. In Alison's case the intention was to harvest her *stem cells*, the key building blocks of the body's immune system, to treat and strengthen them before returning them via a transplant to fight her cancer. Alison was given injections to stimulate her stem cells to enter her bloodstream from her bone marrow; her blood was temporarily withdrawn; the stem cells were extracted from her blood; and the blood then reinfused.

After another high dose of chemotherapy to further reduce the number of cancerous cells in Alison's system, she was ready for her transplant. She had an *autologous transplant*, the process by which a patient receives their own cells back which have been stored since aphaeresis.

The alternative form of stem cell transplant is an *allogeneic transplant*, which is prescribed if the patient's own stem cells are too damaged or are unsuitable to be harvested and effectively restart the immune system. In an allogeneic transplant, stem cells taken from a third-party donor are infused into a patient's bloodstream—at the time of writing allogeneic transplants are carried out more rarely because close tissue-type matches between donor and recipient are so scarce.

In both autologous and allogeneic transplants, the stem cells are introduced into the bloodstream and they then move around the body rebuilding the patient's immune system.

As a stem cell transplant fundamentally restarts the body's immunity from scratch, it places the patient at high risk of infection in its early stages, and has to be carried out in a rigorously controlled environment. For the first ten days or so Alison's family had to don protective masks and gowns to visit her, as did every doctor and nurse involved in her care and treatment, so that the area around her was a germ-free zone. Until her immune system built itself back up, even a simple cold could have had serious consequences. Alison was in hospital for three weeks after the transplant.

Since the transplant Alison has resumed taking Revlimid®—the global trial was deemed a success—and regularly takes vitamin supplements. The bone weakness associated with myeloma often leads to osteoporosis, so she also goes into hospital once every three months as a day patient for a course of Zometa®, a drug that strengthens the bones and delays the onset of osteoporosis. She has monthly blood tests to check her cancer markers.

A cure for myeloma is yet to be found so Alison may well always have the disease, but the combination of treatments she has received since diagnosis means that more than ten years later the condition is being managed effectively. Alison is still teaching maths and science, she has walked across the island of Tasmania with her daughter, and she has written a memoir about her cancer experience.

———

Immunotherapy harnesses the body's own defences to overcome cancer. The immune system needs some assistance to fight cancer because the majority of cancer cells are not different enough to normal cells in their make-up to be recognised as harmful, while those cells the immune system does identify as harmful are often too strong to be destroyed.

*Non-specific immunotherapy* involves injections that give a general boost to the body's immune system, strengthening it in its fight against all types of disease and infection, including cancers.

The biggest breakthroughs in cancer treatment in the last few years, however, have been the development of specific immunotherapies that target individual proteins in cancer cells. The development of these immunotherapies has been made possible by great advances in the understanding of the science of tumour development and behaviour.

The American *Science* magazine reported in December 2013 that the 'new approach to cancer treatment that harnesses the body's own immunity to overcome cancer' is revolutionary. By targeting the body's own defences, as opposed to traditional treatment aimed at attacking the cancerous tumour, the journal described immunotherapy as a 'paradigm shift' in cancer treatment.

# NOT A NEW SCIENCE

Immunotherapy is not a new science. The ability of the body's own immune system to fight cancer was actually first recognised back in 1892 when William Coley, a surgeon at the Memorial Hospital in New York City, observed that some of his cancer patients got better when they developed infections in hospital—their immune systems cranked up to fight the infections and as a result their tumours reduced. As a result of this discovery, and tests he conducted on them, injecting cancer patients with bacteria to bring on infections was adopted and used as a form of treatment for many years, albeit with varying degrees of success.

But advances in surgical techniques and radiotherapy in the 1930s led to them being the most popular and invested-in forms of treatment, and the use of bacteria to bolster the immune system became a backwater.

## MacFarlane Burnet

The intellectual father of modern immunotherapy is MacFarlane Burnet. He won a Nobel Prize for laying out a basic understanding of transplant graft acceptance, the process by which a patient's immune system can be treated to prevent it from rejecting a donor organ that has been transplanted. Without intervention the immune system will reject donor organs as an alien body, in the same way that it fights infections borne by foreign bacteria and viruses.

This idea, revealed in an article in the *British Medical Journal* in 1957, was the first time anyone had highlighted the fact that cancer cells are highly mutated, and that cancer survives because a patient's immune system becomes tolerant to it. Burnet identified a pathway for researchers: 'What is to be sought,' he said at the time, 'is some means whereby the protective mechanism of the body has its reactivity against minor deviations from self-patterns made more sensitive, the converse of the effect of cortisone in damping down immunological reactivity.' (Cortisone suppresses the immune system.)

### Developing Burnet's theories

Burnet's theories were adopted and developed in the laboratory, and in the last decade, due to the work of people such as Mark Smyth and Jim Allison, they have become reality.

According to Professor Jonathan Cebon, what Burnet was envisaging is exactly what we now have in the clinic and on the market through pharmacies—immune-oncology drugs that act as a converse to cortisone, freeing the immune system and encouraging it to fight the cancer.

Professor Cebon says that until relatively few years ago if someone walked through his door with metastatic melanoma they could expect to be dead within six to twelve months. 'That was the general outcome of patients with Stage 4 melanoma,' he explains. 'That outlook has changed dramatically in the last five years because of two areas of treatment that have evolved very dramatically—targeted therapies and immunotherapies.

'In 1990,' Professor Cebon continues, 'the one-year survival chance of a Stage 4 melanoma patient was less than 30%, and the probability of them still being alive two years later was less—below 15%. In 2015, 80–85% of patients are still alive one year after diagnosis of the disease.'

## STEM CELL TRANSPLANTS

Bone marrow and stem cell transplants are forms of *adoptive cell transfer*—a type of immunotherapy in which T cells (a type of immune cell) are given to a patient to help the body fight diseases, such as cancer—that are used to boost the immune systems of blood cancer patients and patients with other forms of cancer whose immune systems have been affected by radiotherapy or chemotherapy treatment.

In an *autologous transfer*, doctors take healthy white blood cells out of a patient, then grow them in a controlled environment in the lab much quicker and in greater number than would naturally happen in the body. The healthy cells are then reintroduced into the patient and travel through the circulatory system to the affected part of the body, where they attach themselves to, and attack, the cancerous cells.

This form of adoptive cell transfer—the one that Alison underwent—is the safest form because it involves removing, treating and then reintroducing a patient's own cells back into their body.

The alternative, an *allogeneic* transfer, uses donor cells from a third party and carries the risk that the patient's immune system will develop *graft versus host disease* (GVHD). This means that because the host's immune system does not recognise the donor cells' DNA, the body rejects the donor cells. For this reason the best donor is a family member because their DNA is close to that of the patient. A twin sibling is regarded as the best possible donor, as they will have the closest DNA match. However, having a family donor does not guarantee success. Similarly, not having a family donor does not necessarily mean the new cells will be rejected.

Doctors prefer an autologous transfer because of the risk of GVHD, but this is only successful if the patient has enough healthy white cells. Doctors cannot grow new, effective cells if the patient's blood is too badly affected, in which case they need healthier donor cells.

GVHD can be treated in some cases. However, a mild form of the disease can actually be beneficial as the donor cells are also attacking the patient's cancer cells when they attack the new cells.

## SIGNALLING THERAPIES

The key to immunotherapy is identifying the individual parts of a cell that make it 'go rogue' and become cancerous.

'Cancer cells are complicated balls of molecules,' Professor Cebon explains, 'and there are signals that get sent from one molecule to another. When mutations take place within the DNA, abnormal signalling develops within the cell. That abnormal signalling can drive the growth of the cell. In melanoma the commonest mutation which takes place—in 40% to 50% of patients—is a molecule called BRAF. This molecule is responsible for conducting a message down into the nucleus of the cell, which instructs the cell to grow, survive and divide.

'The impact the abnormality has on how the cell behaves depends on the dominance of the gene that is mutating,' Professor Cebon explains. 'A *passenger mutation* is an abnormality that does not affect the way a cell behaves, whereas a *driver mutation* will cause the cell to subdivide and grow in an uncontrolled fashion, creating a tumour. The challenge is to figure out whether a detected abnormality is a driver of the tumour. Mutations in RAS proteins, RAF proteins and various other proteins usually result in tumour development.'

*RAS proteins* are essential in the behaviour of individual cells, and *RAF proteins* transmit signals between cells in the pathway that controls their growth and proliferation.

'The response to BRAF inhibitors shows how important it is to identify the right target,' Professor Cebon says. 'If you can find the right target you can block it and have a big impact on the disease. But if you can't work out what the right target is, you don't know what to block and you cannot, therefore, treat the disease. The focus in the coming years is to develop diagnostics: not just to interrogate the DNA of the tumour, which is a huge task, but to pull out from all that information the little piece that tells you which mutation is driving the tumour.

'The DNA is made up of genes, genes produce proteins, and proteins are what determine the biology of the cell,' Professor Cebon continues. 'If you have a damaged gene, that will result in a damaged protein, and a damaged protein can affect the normal behaviour of the cell. The protein may be damaged in a way that doesn't make a difference—a *passenger*—but it can drive the development of a tumour.

'BRAF is like a little engine,' he says. 'When it is behaving normally it can be switched on and off, but when it mutates it gets jammed in the "on" position, like someone tying a weight to the accelerator pedal of the car so it is constantly revving. In the case of BRAF this means it is constantly pushing the cell to subdivide and, therefore, growing the tumour. If you use a drug to block the action of the BRAF, you can have a significant impact on the outcome for the patient.'

Professor Cebon tells a story that graphically illustrates just how significant this impact can be. 'I had a 27-year-old,' he says, 'who walked through the door with a liver full of secondary tumours. Three months later, after his BRAF was blocked, his liver is almost back to normal—the tumours have melted away because the BRAF has not been there driving them on.'

Wider statistics confirm that this was not a one-off event. In a recent clinical trial of a BRAF inhibitor the tumours completely disappeared in over 10% of patients; two-thirds of patients saw their tumours reduced in size by 30% or more; in the remainder of patients the tumour stayed the same or grew.

'The result of the trial means that in the last group there was more than one driver causing their cancer,' says Professor Cebon. 'BRAF was not the only gene which had mutated. The cell is very complex, and if there are a lot of mutations taking place you do not necessarily solve the problem by dealing with the most dominant gene mutation. Although in that final group there was a BRAF mutation—and the adverse effect of that was curtailed by the BRAF inhibitor drug—other mutations took over once the BRAF was neutralised, which became drivers themselves and kept the tumour growing.'

BRAF inhibitor therapy is one of the poster children of targeted therapies. The problem with it, according to Professor Cebon—as in the case of the young man whose liver tumours were almost completely wiped out in three months—is that its effects begin to wear off after six to nine months. The next challenge for researchers is to try and develop therapies with longer-lasting effects.

## IMMUNE SURVEILLANCE

Despite capturing the popular imagination, Burnet's 1957 hypothesis that tumours could be recognised and eliminated by the immune system—a process he called *immune surveillance*—did not catch on with the medical establishment. As a result, there was very little focus on immunology in cancer treatment until very recently. The only exception is bone marrow transplants, which have been used since the 1960s in the treatment of leukaemia.

Professor Cebon tells another story that confirms the power of the immune system and our vulnerability when it is not able to fully function.

'Ten years ago a person who needed a transplant was given a kidney from a seemingly healthy donor,' he says. 'When the kidney failed it was removed and found to be full of malignant melanoma. When they went back into the medical history of the donor they discovered that he had had a melanoma 16 years previously. Those melanoma cells had existed in the body of someone who on the face of it was healthy, and only became apparent when the organ was transplanted into the body of a patient who had been given strong drugs to suppress their immune system, so it did not reject the donor kidney.

'This shows that immune surveillance works,' says Professor Cebon, 'as these cancer cells were held in check by a normal immune system, but were able to re-emerge when introduced into an environment in which the immune system was suppressed.'

## REGULATORY CELLS

'In Stage 4 melanoma there has always been a small proportion of patients who have defied the odds and survive for 15 years or more,' Professor Cebon says. 'Tests show that what these patients have in common is a high number of lymphocytes in their tumours.'

*Lymphocytes* are white blood cells of the immune system, and when they are able to infiltrate cancers they are known as *tumour infiltrating lymphocytes*.

'Today people suffering from bowel, breast and most other forms of cancer who have these tumour infiltrating lymphocytes in their cancers are showing much better outcomes,' Professor Cebon says. 'This implies that an activated immune system inside the cancer is important in holding the tumour back from growing.'

He acknowledges that there is still much to learn about these regulatory cells before they can be fully exploited, and potentially replicated in the laboratory to be developed as *monoclonal antibodies*—laboratory-made proteins that mimic our body's immune system to help fight off harmful pathogens—that can be used as therapy.

'It is not yet clear why these lymphocytes are present in some people and not in others, and in some tumours and not in others, so that is the focus of research happening now,' Professor Cebon says.

## KILLER T CELLS

Cytotoxic T cells are the immune system's weapons against disease, able to recognise and kill virally infected and cancerous cells in the body. They patrol the body looking for targets.

'T cells move through body tissue by pushing out the membrane at the leading edge of the cell and pulling themselves forward,' explains Professor Cebon. 'When a T cell encounters a cancer cell an explosion of membrane protrusions explores the surface of the target. The T cells then kill the cancer cell with toxic granules that are secreted directly into the target, protecting innocent bystanders nearby. As the membrane of the target is compromised by the toxins in the granules, the cancer cell dies.

'This process takes place on a cell-by-cell basis, and an active immune system will work through a tumour, killing as many cells as it finds.

'However,' he says, 'the immune system does not operate incessantly—it is switched on and off. The switch is triggered by particular molecules immune cells recognise on cells they meet as they move around the body—when they meet a molecule they recognise as being "bad", they switch themselves on and destroy it; if they meet a molecule on a healthy cell they switch off, and keep moving around quietly until they meet a new "bad" molecule.'

## CO-STIMULATORY MOLECULES AND CHECKPOINT INHIBITORS

The molecules that drive the immune system are known as *co-stimulatory molecules*.

As Professor Cebon explains, 'It is not enough to recognise a cell against which action needs to be taken; a message also has to be sent through to that effect. Once the body's immune system recognises a cell that is harmful and that needs to be targeted, the co-stimulatory molecules act as accelerators, or *amplifiers*, which stimulate the necessary action to be taken against the offending cell.

'The molecules which prevent any action being taken, in essence the "off switches", are called *checkpoints*,' Professor Cebon adds. 'Checkpoint inhibitors are drugs which interfere with the checkpoint and reverse the message it sends that "there's nothing to see here, no action needed". All tissues need to control immune reaction against themselves, and that is why checkpoints are a necessary part of the body, but they allow cancer cells to survive by preventing the immune system taking action against them. Checkpoint inhibitors allow the immune system to see through that "disguise" and attack the cancer cells.'

*Checkpoint inhibitors* are proteins that prevent the immune system from harming the healthy tissue. Cancers have developed a way of hiding the threat they pose, and fooling the checkpoint inhibitors into stopping the immune system deploying T cells to attack the cancer.

Jim Allison is seen as the pioneer of modern immunotherapy as a result of his work to identify a protein called CTLA-4 that works as a checkpoint, preventing the body's immune system from attacking cancer cells. Allison and his team developed an antibody to block the CTLA-4 protein on the immune system's 'killer' T cells, releasing them to attack tumours. The antibody was developed into a drug, ipilimumab, that was approved by the FDA in the USA for the treatment of metastatic melanoma in 2011. It has had unprecedented results for many melanoma patients whose cancer has spread far and wide, including to the brain.

Subsequently researchers have identified and managed to create an antibody called PD-1 for another checkpoint. Like CTLA-4 inhibitors, it was initially developed to treat advanced melanoma, but is now also proving successful in trials for patients with other forms of cancer.

'Understanding the molecular brakes and accelerators is the breakthrough that has enabled drugs to be developed that manipulate immunity,' explains Professor Cebon. 'A clinical trial for Stage 4 melanoma patients reported in 2014 that a PD-1 inhibitor combined with a CTLA-4 inhibitor shrank the tumours of over 50% of patients taking part to virtually nothing within 10 to 12 weeks. In some patients the tumours stopped growing, and in only three patients the tumours continued growing. This trial saw 82% of patients being alive one year after developing Stage 4 melanoma, and over 70% of them still alive three years later.

'That trial was just one cancer type with the first two immunotherapy drugs off the assembly line,' he says. 'There are now dozens of immune-regulating drugs being developed by pharmaceutical companies, and medical professionals are working out how to manipulate the immune system and how to select patients more effectively.'

Clinical trials are now being conducted not just for melanoma patients, but also for people with lung, kidney and bladder cancer and an ever-growing number of conditions. It is believed that ultimately immunotherapies could be successful against all types of cancer.

'Going forward, we will work on combinations of immunotherapy drugs, figuring out how to individualise therapy,' Professor Cebon says. 'Just as you need to find a MEK [a gene that transmits chemical signals to cells] mutation or a BRAF mutation to identify the patient who is best going to respond to a BRAF inhibitor, we believe it should be possible to characterise the inflammation within the tumour and answer the question, "Which immunotherapy, or combination of immunotherapies, might work most effectively for these patients?" This could significantly improve survival rates, not just in melanoma but in other cancers as well.'

◆ ◆ ◆

Professor Cebon concludes that the potential of immunotherapy today is reminiscent of the advances in combination chemotherapy in the 1950s that dramatically changed life expectancy for people with childhood leukaemia and Hodgkin's lymphoma. Hodgkin's today has a survival rate of over 90% in the first year after diagnosis, and more than 80% of patients are still alive 10 years after developing the condition.

'I am not saying that we will find a cure for cancer in the next 10 years,' says Professor Cebon. 'But I really do believe that the developments in immunotherapy, in particular, will mean that the cancer landscape will be very different a decade from now.'

## Chapter 7

# IMPROVING THE OUTCOMES COMBINATION TREATMENTS

Traditionally, a cancer diagnosis was usually followed by an operation, a number of sessions of radiotherapy and/or a course of chemotherapy. Each treatment was carried out separately, appraising the success of one before another was prescribed. Today, a combination of two or more types of treatment is delivered simultaneously to provide a more intense, coordinated attack on the cancerous cells and reduce treatment time.

In this chapter we will discover:

◆ which treatment types are used in conjunction with each other

◆ why these combine successfully

◆ how these combinations improve outcomes.

Let's begin with Louisa's success story.

## From horror story to happy ending

Louisa was 31 years old when she was diagnosed with breast cancer. After living in London for two and a half years, she first noticed something amiss when she returned to Melbourne for Christmas in 2008.

'My friend Mary and I were sitting on the beach at Lorne,' she said. 'I was putting sunscreen on and I noticed that I had a lump here on the side and quite big. And I thought, I can't ignore that.

'But I was 31 and not for one second did I worry that it was cancer; I was incredibly ignorant about the fact that younger women can get cancer—I thought you had to be at least 50. And I didn't think it was worth remarking on.'

Louisa made an appointment with her London GP about a week after she got back. She had so much work to catch up on at her publishing job that she didn't want to take more time off for a doctor's appointment.

'It was February by then. The GP said, "It's probably nothing, but it's NHS policy to send you to the breast clinic just in case." I remember thinking later, thank God they've got that policy because he and I wouldn't have done anything.'

She went to have a biopsy a couple of weeks later. 'The specialist said she thought it was something called a *breast mouse*, which is some kind of benign mass.'

Louisa made an appointment to get her results during her lunchbreak, several days later. 'I'd left my computer on as I was going to jump on the bus, get my results and come back.'

Kings College Hospital in South London is a teaching hospital. When a surgeon called Louisa in, he had a med student with him.

'He started saying, "Okay so you went to your GP and he sent you here," and I thought at one point, why is he narrating my story back to me? Something alarmed me about that. And I was on my own—I hadn't brought a friend with me.

'And he said, "So you had the biopsy and we have the results and the results are you have cancer. You will have to have chemotherapy, you will lose your breast or both your breasts and you will lose your hair." This is how he said it to me: bang, bang, bang, as though I was being shot. And there was this kid sitting there and I'm just going wait, what's happening, just total shock. It was just like, don't sugarcoat it.

'In a way it's better to just tell people, but I was totally unprepared; it was like a bolt out of the blue. If I'd been older or had some history of it or been expecting it, I would have taken a friend with me, but I couldn't have predicted what they were going to say to me so it was just like being sideswiped. So then I just burst into tears—I was totally panicked and shocked—and then they organised for me to talk to a breast-care nurse.'

Louisa rang the office to say she wasn't coming back that day and asked them to turn her computer off. 'I'd thought I was going to be an hour max.'

Louisa took her nurse friend Steve to the appointment with the breast-care nurse. 'And she was fabulous, I think if she'd been the one to deliver the news it would have been more sensitively put.'

Steve was great to have as a support person. When he had to go Louisa rang some other friends, but then she had to catch the bus home to her flat alone. 'My flatmate was going out and she said, "Do you want me to cancel?" and I said no; I really just wanted to be on my own. After she left I remember just grabbing my pillow and screaming into it, it was so bizarre, and then I had to ring Mum and Dad and I think it was their morning.

'That was the worst because then you have to wait—there's a period of time between the diagnosis and the prognosis and you don't know if they're going to tell you you've got cancer through your whole body and you're going to die. It's like your life's on hold.'

The night after she found out, she had arranged to take her guitar to a pub and perform some songs at a friend's 30th. 'So that day I decided that I was going to do it. When I got to Steve's place I said "Guess what?" as I started to walk into his kitchen, and he said "What?" and I said "I'm going to be fine, I just have to have the treatment" and he said [Irish accent], "I've been waiting for you to figure that out."

'So I just had to have 24 hours of this oh my God I'm gonna die, and then I came out of it, it was like being underwater and coming up for air and going, potentially I'm fine, you just have to go through and follow the steps.

'When I had the surgery they took lymph nodes out to check—I had a lumpectomy and didn't have to lose a breast. But it was lucky, they said the tumour hadn't spread anywhere; it was about three and a half centimetres. And then you think—if I'd waited another week it probably would have been making its way elsewhere.'

After the surgery, Louisa returned to Australia and had 'just in case' chemo at Melbourne's Peter MacCallum Cancer Centre—they'd taken the tumour, but some rogue cells may have remained somewhere—and then radiation, localised in the same area to make sure no cancer could survive.

'The side effects of chemo weren't too bad,' she commented. 'I was really lucky because my breast cancer was hormone-negative. If it had been positive, that's when they give you tamoxifen. So when I was done I was done, whereas friends of mine have been having to take tamoxifen for years and that's got its own side effects.'

Louisa also tested negative to BRCA1 and BRCA2 gene mutations—brought to international attention by actor-activist-filmmaker Angelina Jolie—which increase the lifetime risk of breast and ovarian cancers. 'So everything post diagnosis was the best-case scenario.'

Louisa has since married and recovered fully—carefully monitored by brief annual mammogram and ultrasound check-ups. 'There's always a risk it can affect your fertility,' she said. Yet, although she had frozen some eggs, she became pregnant naturally with her first baby, Feehan, in 2016. The breast that had treatment produced milk, but much less.

When it came time to give Feehan a sibling, she used some frozen eggs. Again, she was able to breastfeed for a few months, but supply was an issue.

Now Dashiell is one, Louisa is fully occupied between two energetic little boys and part-time teaching work.

---

Today, treatment often involves a combination of two or more types of treatment simultaneously:

◆ radiotherapy or chemotherapy being administered during surgery

◆ delivery of chemotherapy during a session of radiotherapy

◆ doses of different chemotherapy drugs given at the same time.

## SURGERY COMBINATIONS

### Combining surgery and chemotherapy

Usually chemotherapy is delivered via a syringe through the patient's skin and into the body's network of blood vessels—a process known as *systematic chemotherapy*.

Administering chemotherapy directly into cancerous cells—taking advantage of the access to tumours that surgery offers—enables a higher concentration of chemotherapy to be used because the risk of damage to healthy parts of the body is removed, as well as to the circulatory system, through which the drugs normally have to travel to reach the tumour.

*Hyperthermic intraperitoneal chemotherapy* (HIPEC) significantly enhances the effectiveness of surgery to remove tumours from the abdominal cavity by delivering a concentrated dose of chemotherapy to the area immediately after the actual procedure, while the patient is still anaesthetised and the abdominal area open and accessible.

The drug solution used for HIPEC is heated, which increases its rate of absorption into the tumour tissue. This is another benefit that systematic chemotherapy cannot offer, as the higher temperature of the drugs cannot be maintained once they enter the bloodstream. HIPEC targets microscopic cancer cells that remain in the body after tumour-removal surgery, reducing the chances of the cancer recurring.

This process is used in the treatment of primary cancers of the bowel, colon, appendix and ovaries, and secondary tumours that spread to the abdomen from other parts of the body.

## Combining surgery and radiotherapy

A tumour-removal operation very rarely succeeds in removing every single cancerous cell from the body. There are usually microscopic malignant cells that have spread beyond the main tumour being targeted by the surgeon, or are left behind because they are 'hiding' behind an organ or a larger piece of healthy tissue. Because it is so difficult to remove every vestige of a tumour, many cancer patients see a recurrence of their condition, often months after seemingly successful surgery.

A course of post-operative radiation, historically prescribed after surgery in cancers prone to recurrence, has a couple of drawbacks:

◆ It usually cannot start for some time as the body needs to heal after the surgery, giving the microscopic cancer cells left behind a chance to re-establish themselves.

◆ Post-operative courses of radiotherapy often involve up to five sessions of treatment a week for up to a couple of months.

*Intraoperative radiation therapy* (IORT) delivers a dose of radiation to the area around a tumour during the surgery being carried out to remove it. Administering the radiation during surgery means it does not have to pass through healthy tissue, and nearby sensitive areas can be shielded or moved out of the way during the procedure, so a higher dose of radiation can be delivered to the target area. The probability of the cancer recurring is reduced, as the microscopic cancerous cells usually left behind are killed by the radiation, and the need for weeks of post-operative radiotherapy is less likely.

*Intraperitoneal chemotherapy* (IP) is a combination of surgery and chemotherapy that is used to treat ovarian cancer patients whose cancer has reached an advanced stage, but that has not spread beyond the abdomen. IP is administered via a catheter which is placed into the abdominal cavity during cytoreductive surgery to reduce the size of their tumour, or specifically to deliver the chemotherapy using a *laparoscopy* (keyhole surgery). This method delivers a high dose of chemotherapy directly to the tumour, but has the added advantage of that some of the drug is absorbed into the bloodstream from where it reaches cancer cells that have spread beyond the site of the original tumour.

## CHEMOTHERAPY COMBINATIONS

### Combining chemotherapy and radiotherapy

*Chemoradiation*, a combination of chemotherapy and radiotherapy administered in the same treatment session, is being used increasingly in the fight against a range of different cancers. Results indicate that in many cases the two methods of treatment are more effective when combined than when given in separate courses one after the other. It is believed this is because the chemotherapy weakens the defences of the cancer and makes it more vulnerable to the effects of the radiation therapy.

In some cases, chemoradiation is used to shrink a tumour prior to surgery to remove it, but the combination treatment can also be effective instead of surgery, in cases where an operation is neither possible nor likely to be successful. As with combination chemotherapy, chemoradiation enables doctors to attack the cancer with a higher intensity without causing unbearable side effects for the patient: because chemotherapy and radiotherapy have different effects they can be used at the same time. Most patients receiving chemoradiation do so as day patients, able to return home after a few hours of treatment.

This approach is used most commonly in the treatment of head and neck cancers, oesophageal cancer and bowel cancer, but clinical trials of combinations of chemotherapy and radiotherapy in the treatment of many other cancers are taking place regularly.

In September 2014 a team at the University of Pittsburgh Medical Center announced a breakthrough in the treatment of pancreatic cancer involving a combination of chemotherapy and radiotherapy. The only actual cure for pancreatic cancer is surgery to remove the tumour, but this particular cancer is often at an advanced stage by the time it is diagnosed and, in many cases, surgery is no longer possible.

The trial combined a course of chemotherapy followed immediately by three treatments of SABR, which is detailed in Chapter 4, Radiotherapy. The tumours of almost half of the patients who took part in the trial had shrunk to the point that surgeons were able to operate on them, and 90% of those who had surgery did not experience any recurrence of their cancer in the year after the procedure.

A phase II clinical trial was conducted in the US in 2017. The team reported that combining radiation therapy with chemotherapy for some patients with limited metastatic NSCLC slowed their disease significantly compared to NSCLC patients who only received chemotherapy. Another research team revealed at the same time that adding radiation to chemotherapy helped patients with metastatic colorectal cancer and sarcoma.

Today, combining radiotherapy and chemotherapy has become widespread when treating many locally advanced diseases.

### *Combining chemotherapies*

Using a combination of drugs at the same time has been effective in reducing the capability of cancers to develop resistance to chemotherapy. Using one drug followed by another allows cancerous cells time to become resistant to each, whereas trials have shown cells cannot resist two different drugs simultaneously—if the cells develop resistance to one drug, then the other will kill them off.

The key aim of chemotherapy is to interrupt metastasis, by which cancer cells rapidly grow and divide. Metastasis takes place in stages, and using different drugs that simultaneously target more than one stage of the process has been shown to be effective against cancers that are too strong or fast-acting to be stopped by single-drug treatments. Combining one agent that attacks the cancer cell's DNA with another that interferes with their ability to rapidly divide greatly reduces the ability of cancer cells to resist the treatment.

For example, a couple of forms of ovarian cancer are treated with a combination of three drugs. Patients with *germ cell tumours,* which originate in the egg cells in the ovary, or *stromal tumours,* a rarer form that develops in the hormone-producing tissue within the ovaries, often receive a combination called BEP. This treatment involves patients receiving a combination of the three drugs over three-day cycles. They are bleomycin, an antibiotic that interferes with the rapid growth of cancer cells; etoposide, a drug that impacts on the DNA of the cancerous cells; and a platinum-based compound, one of the mainstays in the treatment of all forms of ovarian cancer.

It is often not possible to maximise the effectiveness of chemotherapy treatment with very high doses of one particular drug, due to the side effects for the patient. As different drugs have different effects, using more than one allows a more intense overall dose of combined chemotherapy to be used at the same time, increasing the impact of the treatment.

Combination chemotherapy is proving to be particularly effective in the palliative treatment of advanced, incurable cancers, reducing the severity of the symptoms for the patient and increasing their life expectancy.

### Combining chemotherapy and immunotherapy

Chemotherapy is increasingly being supplemented with immunotherapies to improve its effectiveness. This is a new phenomenon in the second decade of the 2000s and contradicts the previously-held view among medical experts around the world that the two types of treatment are not compatible: chemotherapy drugs are designed to kill cells and reduce immunity, whereas the whole point behind immunotherapy is to empower cells to fix themselves.

Some cancers are resistant to both chemotherapy and immunotherapy when either of those treatment types are administered in isolation. The most recent research reveals that these cells are weakened when the two approaches are used together. Using immunotherapy checkpoint inhibitors to block the activity of specific proteins in cancer cells has allowed certain chemotherapy drugs to be far more effective than when they were used by themselves.

For example, a study concluded in 2018 found that some patients suffering from advanced melanoma, who had not responded to immune checkpoint inhibitors as a sole treatment type, began to benefit from them when they were used in conjunction with local chemotherapy. And in 2019 a professor of medical oncology at Rush University Medical College wrote a paper urging medical teams to use a combination of immunotherapy and chemotherapy as the first-line treatment for both patients with NSCLC and small cell lung cancer whose tumours had developed to a certain stage. Their research suggests that the combination could be effective for all patients with either of those cancers.

A number of clinical trials now taking place around the world show that the combination of chemotherapy and immunotherapy could play a major role in the future treatment of a range of cancers. Initial results have been particularly encouraging in combinations designed to fight pancreatic cancer, a form of blood cancer called *chronic lymphocytic leukaemia*, and metastatic prostate cancer.

## IMMUNOTHERAPY COMBINATIONS

### *Combining radiotherapy and immunotherapy*
Research conducted in the last five years has revealed that radiation of cancer cells can bring about a chemical reaction that makes them more vulnerable to attack by immunotherapy drugs. These effects

are not only immediate but can also be long-term, producing a form of immune memory that increases the chances of the body fighting recurrence of the cancer after months or even years of dormancy.

This development in our knowledge of how radiation can be harnessed to treat cancer is significant because it is the first time that radiotherapy can be used to stimulate cells to behave in a different way, as opposed to its usual aim of eliminating cells. A number of clinical trials are now taking place around the world into the effects of combined radiotherapy and immunotherapy. Increasing evidence shows that the two are mutually beneficial: given the right level of radiation, radiotherapy can improve positive responses to checkpoint inhibitors; similarly, tumours that have been treated with immunotherapy drugs are less resistant to radiotherapy.

The ongoing research suggests that combining radiotherapy and immunotherapy will play an important role in the treatment of, and improve the outcome for, patients with various forms of advanced cancer, who have already gone through long periods of other forms of treatment.

### Combining immunotherapies

One of the body's most important protein groups is the *inhibitors of apoptosis* (IAP) proteins, which play a central role in the immune system's ability to fight cancer. IAP proteins regulate the cycle of cell regeneration and are involved in the dying out of cells that have fulfilled their normal function.

An *oncolytic virus* is a naturally occurring virus that is predisposed to attack cancer cells. Since the early 2000s geneticists around the world have been conducting research into these viruses to find a way that they can be safely and effectively harnessed for cancer treatment.

Initial trials of IAP and oncolytic viruses as stand-alone cancer treatments showed promise, with some early studies finding that when IAP proteins were combined with an oncolytic virus, the rate at which tumours can be destroyed increased dramatically compared to when they are used singly. Subsequent research into IAPs has hit some hurdles: their toxic nature and inconclusive results in terms of their efficacy has prevented the development of therapies for widespread clinical use as yet. However, research is ongoing and advances in medicinal biochemistry and the understanding of *biomarkers*—molecules that reveal whether or not processes in cells are normal or abnormal and, therefore, whether or not disease is present—means that effective apoptosis-targeted agents could well be available in the near future.

◆ ◆ ◆

The very nature of cancer means that cells constantly change as they mutate, so they are adept at building up a resistance to individual treatment types.

Previously the medical profession attempted one form of treatment, and waited to see its effect before moving on to another. This enabled cancer to 'come to grips' with the individual weapon being used against it, and it could then move on to deal with whatever was thrown at it next.

Using the increased understanding of the different processes that sustain cancer—and targeting them simultaneously with multiple approaches—is leading to better results for patients.

# Chapter 8

# MAKING IT PERSONAL PERSONALISED MEDICINE AND CANCER GENOMICS

Personalised medicine represents a fundamental shift in the approach to dealing with cancer. Breakthroughs in this field mean that today two people with the same form of cancer and experiencing similar symptoms may well be given different treatment, based on what their genes indicate will work for them.

Now we will discover how personalised medicine is helping:

◆ understand why and how cancer develops

◆ work out which treatments will be effective for each individual

◆ predict what diseases a person is likely to develop in future.

Personalised medicine focuses on each patient's own genetic make-up, rather than the type of cancer they are suffering from. Everyone's genes are different, and the research behind personalised medicine involves the study of how an individual will react to a particular drug.

This field of research is called *genomics*—the examination of the complete set of genetic information you have, which determines how your body functions and what it looks like.

Now it is known that two or more cancers in different parts of one person's body will often have the same genetic mutation, both cancers can be treated in the same way, whereas in the past a different drug for each form of cancer would have been prescribed.

◆ ◆ ◆

Professor David Bowtell, then Head of Cancer Genomics and Genetics at Melbourne's Peter MacCallum Cancer Centre, calls personalised medicine the future of cancer treatment. So, to get a clearer understanding of what is a complex area, we spoke to Professor Bowtell about the role our genetic make-up plays in our susceptibility to developing cancer, and how it can be harnessed to fight the condition.

## UNDERSTANDING CANCER THROUGH GENETICS

Every organism has a genome that contains all the information needed to create it, maintain it as a living entity and enable it to reproduce. A human's genome is made up of three billion base pairs of DNA, and the nucleus of every cell in the body contains a copy of the code. Every thousand or so bases, there's one base difference between each individual, which makes each genome unique.

Professor Bowtell likens our genome to the operating system of a laptop. 'Imagine that you have billions of laptops all running Mac OS—that is what our genome is like, billions of cells all running the same operating system.'

The *germline* is the population of cells in our body that is involved in reproduction, and it is passed on from generation to generation. Any mutations in germline cells are *hereditary*—not the result of environmental factors we experience or lifestyle choices we make. We inherit them from our parents and pass them on to our children irrespective of where or how we live.

*Germline genetics* governs the susceptibility each of us has to developing cancer. As Professor Bowtell explains: 'Some people are born with mutations in their operating system that increase their likelihood of developing cancer, either a little or a lot.' Our germline is inherited from our mother and father: those of us who carry mutations in genes that have a profound impact on whether we develop cancer tend to be from families that have a history of a lot of cancer down the generations.

People with mutations in genes that play a key role in suppressing tumours have a high risk of developing cancer. For example, a mutation in BRCA1 or BRCA2 genes significantly increases the risk of developing breast cancer or ovarian cancer; a mutation in the P16 gene heightens the danger of melanoma; and a mutation of the APC gene leads to a higher chance of rapid cell growth and division in the lower intestines and, therefore, a greater risk of colorectal cancer.

There are many other genes where the mutations slightly modify the behaviour of the protein in the cell, and therefore what the cell does. 'Mutations in these low-risk genes can increase your chances of developing cancer a little bit, and whether or not you go on to develop cancer depends on how many of these mutations you have,' says Professor Bowtell. 'One really bad mutation might be enough to give you cancer; a couple of minor ones might not make any difference; but half a dozen or more even really small ones can synergise and be a big risk.'

### Nature and nurture

Professor Bowtell emphasises that although our germline genetics govern our predisposition to cancer, they do not categorically define whether or not we will get it. The interaction between genes and the environment is vital.

'If you're fair-skinned and fair-haired, that increases your chance of developing skin cancer: if you live in a sunny place with lots of UV you're far more likely to end up with a melanoma; but if you live somewhere where the sun rarely shines, or if you cover yourself up all the time, you should be okay,' he says.

This interaction between genome and environment is particularly influential in early life—statistics show that British people who migrated to Australia when they were already in their late twenties or older very rarely develop skin cancer. However, their children who were born in Australia—or were very young when they moved—are at a far higher risk of getting the disease.

The vast majority of cancer cases are a combination of a mutation in a patient's genome and factors in their environment. In very extreme circumstances cancer may develop in people who have no predisposition towards it in their genome, such as those people living and working in Chernobyl who were exposed to high volumes of radioactive particles that were discharged during the accident at the Ukrainian city's nuclear power plant. People with mutations in tumour-suppressing genes that play a key role in controlling the body's cell regeneration cycle are at high risk of developing cancer even if they maintain a very healthy lifestyle, but they will not inevitably develop cancer symptoms. There are no mutations that guarantee the carrier will develop cancer.

According to Professor Bowtell, someone who has a serious mutation of one of the key tumour-suppressing genes has a risk factor of up to 70% of developing cancer by the age of 80. Cancer is different from other diseases in this way—in neurological conditions such as Huntington's disease, having the mutation of the gene that causes it means that developing the symptoms is inevitable.

Most people carry one or two low-risk mutations in different combinations, and for them lifestyle and environment play a very big part in deciding whether or not they develop cancer. Only a very small percentage of the population have devastating mutations of the key genes in the development of cancer, and they usually have a strong family history of cancer. A similarly small proportion of people have germlines that carry no mutations whatsoever and are, therefore, at a very low risk of developing cancer.

## DECODING THE GENOME

Until recently the human genome was a secret code, hidden from us all. The first successful mapping of a human genome took place in the early 2000s and the process took months. Now, because of technology, it can be done much quicker and for a fraction of the cost. That first successful attempt was the result of the investment of several billions of dollars; in 2010, mapping one genome cost several million dollars and took several weeks to do; today, it can be done within seven days for a few thousand dollars.

Despite the downward trend, the cost of genome mapping will not decrease much further. The process of extracting the information itself is being refined and simplified all the time, but analysing the data produced by a genome mapping takes a great deal of time and expertise. That cost, in terms of man hours, will increase over time with inflation.

The first step in mapping the genome is sequencing it. There are four base letters in a genetic alphabet—A, C, G and T—and each individual's genome is made up of three billion pairs of these bases. Sequencing breaks down them down into the combinations in which they are grouped to form a person's DNA. This enables scientists to identify the genes in the DNA, at which point they try to learn how those genes react to each other to develop the cells in the body and manage their behaviour.

Professor Bowtell explains that to be able to predict how the genes will behave, we need to look at the three billion base pairs of DNA in the human genome in multiple combinations of sequences, to ensure we cover all the possible outcomes of processes that the genome drives.

'There is a whole science around mining this data and interpreting it,' he says. 'We know a lot about how to read it, but there is code embedded in code embedded in code. If you took someone's genome and wrote it down once in seven-point font, it would cover the entire surface of the Melbourne Cricket Ground,' he adds.

In the early days of genome mapping the challenges of interpreting so much data meant that scientists were only able to identify a few key genes that had an obvious effect on an individual's propensity to develop cancer. The first one they became aware of was BRCA, a gene that produces proteins that suppress tumours. When BRCA mutates it no longer produces the protein and cannot, therefore, leaves cells vulnerable to developing cancer. BRCA mutations play a major role in many cases of breast and ovarian cancer, and in men lead to an increased risk of prostate cancer.

'Where there's a mutation in a gene that has a really big effect there are practical things that can be done, such as risk-reducing surgery,' Professor Bowtell says. An example of this is Angelina Jolie, who had a preventative double mastectomy because she learned she had a mutation of her BRCA1 gene.

The advances in technology that have widened scientists' understanding of the genetic code mean it is now possible to identify more genes, including some of those that only have a minor effect but that can still lead to developing cancer. Despite the advances in identifying a larger number of genes that can potentially cause problems, the way in which the information is used practically is something that is still being considered

'If you find low-risk genes, what you do about those is still being figured out,' Professor Bowtell explains. 'You don't want to recommend major surgery for something that is fairly improbable, but neither do you want to just advise somebody there is a risk and let them work it out for themselves.'

Currently the information produced by genome mapping is used for risk management. In lower-risk cases it is just a question of regular screening to check whether or not cancer is developing, and to catch it very early if it does. People whose genetic make-up suggests they are at risk of developing bowel cancer are advised to have frequent colonoscopies, and for those showing a tendency to melanoma, skin screens are relatively simple and inexpensive. In higher-risk cases preventative surgery may be the safest option, such as a mastectomy or *oophorectomy* (removal of the ovaries).

If enough people can have their genome mapped in the future, it will be possible to deliver health services to the public in a more targeted and cost-efficient way. Ideally those with a gene mutation will have diagnostic tests for the condition they are at risk of developing, and the effort and expense of testing can be spared for those whose genome reveals not to be at risk. At the moment all men over the age of 50 are recommended to have their prostate tested, but most of those tests are negative—genomics could be used to identify who really is at risk and should therefore be tested.

Sequencing of genomes is changing cancer medicine. As we identify more and more of the genes that signal the risk of developing cancer, people can get tested. Where risk-reducing regimes are indicated, they can be devised to try and stop them from developing disease.

## Somatic genetics

The germline genetics described earlier in this chapter deals with the genes we inherit from our parents and which are not affected by any external conditions or events. *Somatic genetics*, on the other hand, involves changes to our DNA that happen after we are born, and that are brought about by the environment in which we live or things that happen to us.

A melanoma can be caused by the effect of a bolt of UV light hitting one cell in the skin. The UV light is very energetic and it can actually damage the DNA of that cell. Professor Bowtell warns: 'If the bolt of UV light happens to hit a gene that is crucial to the growth of a cell, it might change the DNA code in a way that produces a protein that makes that cell divide rapidly, or the mutation might knock out a gene that makes a protein that stops the cell from dividing rapidly.'

This is an ongoing process, he explains. 'When you get sunburnt you aren't actually burned—the cells in your skin have picked up a whole lot of damage to their DNA and have done one of two things: either they stop what they're doing and they fix it; or, if there's a lot of damage, they say "You know what, there's too much damage here, we're going to kill ourselves." When your skin peels because of sunburn it is actually a whole lot of cells that have decided there is too much damage and it could be dangerous.'

In essence, the body protects itself from serious harm by sacrificing cells that become damaged—the cells commit suicide for the good of the rest of the body. Problems arise when cells try to mend themselves but don't fix everything. In this case a mutation occurs—the mutation can be innocuous, but it can also hold the potential to drive the development of cancer. That cell is then set on a path of becoming a bad cell, and after a number of years it may pick up another mutation, and those two mutations can make it behave really badly.

'You can see this on your skin,' says Professor Bowtell. 'Patches that are a bit scaly—that's a cell that has undergone division and expanded out, and is on the way to being cancerous. If it gets more damaged as you get older and older it can go from being a *solar keratosis*—a precancerous skin condition caused by excessive exposure to sunlight—to a carcinoma.'

Two further examples illustrate how cancers can develop in different parts of the body as a result of seemingly minor events that change the behaviour of cells and set them on a course to becoming malignant.

'A woman can have an initially harmless HPV virus but it starts to change the cells in the cervix. A Pap smear will reveal that these cells are on the way to becoming cancerous,' Professor Bowtell explains. 'Similarly, a gastroenterologist will analyse a colonoscopy and see that an initially benign polyp growing out from the side of the bowel is potentially dangerous—the *polyp* is a cell that has multiplied and multiplied and multiplied and formed a wart-like structure that, if left long enough, will turn into a full-blown cancer. It will eventually turn around, burrow through the side of the bowel wall, enter the bloodstream, go into the liver and the person ends up with metastatic bowel cancer.'

In all these cases an initial mutation that happens over a period of time builds up, causing a change in the genetic code. In germline genetics one person is born with defects in the code, and another person isn't. Somatic genetics deals with situations in which the code is changed in just one cell through the impact of carcinogens such as cigarette smoke, UV light or poor diet.

Professor Bowtell continues: 'A number of these mutations work together, interact with each other and over time develop from a sequence that is abnormal to one that is very abnormal to one that is cancerous.'

In a lot of cancers, he sees clear evidence that incidence of the disease is lower in the screened population than the unscreened population. 'In the case of the person with the polyp on the side of the bowel, early detection means it can be removed before it has the opportunity to develop into bowel cancer.' He believes the big challenge now for the medical profession is to decide who is most appropriate for screening.

In these cases of acquired changes to the genetic code—as opposed to the germline evidence genome mapping reveals with inherent mutations—it is a case of getting people to understand those lifestyle decisions and environmental conditions that increase the risk of changes to their cell DNA occurring that could bring on cancer. A GP is the most appropriate person to decide when screening is worthwhile, based on what they know about their patient's family, diet and lifestyle.

As the development of cancer takes place over a period of time it does, in most cases, present itself later in life. There is little point in screening men for prostate cancer or women for breast cancer before the age of 50—most cases develop after that age, and a clear screen earlier in life does not mean cancer will not develop at a later date.

Changes to somatic cells are not passed on to the next generation. If we develop a skin cancer due to excessive exposure to sunlight triggering a reaction that causes a melanoma, we will not pass that condition on if we reproduce. A mutation in our germline that makes us susceptible to melanoma, however, will be passed on to our progeny.

## Personalised genetics

In the past, when a tumour was removed it would be cut up and looked at through a microscope to try and infer the behaviour of the cells in that cancer. 'Doing this is like trying to see how a city works from 10,000 feet up,' says Professor Bowtell. 'You are too remote to see what's really going on. To fully understand you have to get down to ground level, and to learn how a cancer's behaving means looking at the genes themselves that have been corrupted.'

DNA sequencing techniques can now be used on individual patients in real time to find out what mutations are causing their cancer. For some of the mutations there are drugs that will target those particular mutations and restore normal cell behaviour.

About half of all patients diagnosed with a melanoma caused by sun exposure have a mutation in a gene called BRAF, which makes a protein that is a key enzyme in making cells divide. Mutations in a particular amino acid of the protein convert it into a slightly different compound that bends the protein and makes it behave in a way it wouldn't normally do.

'Much like pushing a light switch on and leaving it pressed on for a period of time,' says Professor Bowtell, 'it sends a series of "go" messages, which makes the cell divide over and over again. There is a drug that targets the BRAF protein, shutting it down and preventing the rapid cell division from taking place. Sequencing a melanoma patient enables doctors to establish if the BRAF mutation has taken place and, if so, the drug can be prescribed.

'This type of situation illustrates how personalised cancer medicine works—you look inside the cells, into the DNA code, you look at what mutations have occurred and whether any of those mutations are actionable. *Actionable* in this context means that there is a drug available that can affect the mutation that is causing the development of the cancer.'

The fundamental aim of personalised medicine is to accurately predict when a specific drug has a very good chance of being effective for a particular patient, in the context of the way their cancer has developed. Straightforward chemotherapy involves a far more general prescription of a drug, or drugs, that have proved effective against the type of cancer the patient has in a large sample of people who have had that condition.

Professor Bowtell says that for centuries the starting point for cancer treatment has been anatomical. 'This person has breast cancer, that person has prostate cancer, the person over there has kidney cancer, and so on,' he explains. 'Even today, if you are diagnosed with ovarian cancer you are referred to a gynae oncologist, if you have lung cancer you go to see a thoracic surgeon, and so on.'

The research into genomics has brought about the realisation within the medical profession that this anatomical approach is quite misleading.

'Metastatic cells remember their heritage,' says Professor Bowtell, 'so the cell in a cancer that starts in the bowel and then spreads to the liver still remembers that it's a bowel cell, and behaves as such. A cell's heritage is written in the way they use the code. When you fire up your laptop you don't run everything—Excel, Word, PowerPoint, your browser and so on—all at the same time, you just open up what you need for the particular task you are doing.

'In the same way a neuron in the brain may never divide in 20 years, whereas a T lymphocyte in the blood divides every six hours: they both have exactly the same code, but they are using it differently, running different parts of the program because they have to specialise. Cells in different parts of the body go under a very complex process of refinement as to how they use the code to achieve what they need to do, so a bowel cell locks in a particular pattern of using the code and that doesn't change even if the cell relocates as part of a metastasising tumour to a different part of the body.'

'Nevertheless,' he adds, 'the classification of cancers is not black and white.'

Ovarian cancer is not necessarily caused by cells that come from the ovary itself. Most fatal ovarian cancers actually come from cells in the *distal fallopian tube*, a catcher's net that catches the egg around the ovary. The biology of the cell, and therefore of the cancer, is different to that of a cell from the ovary itself.

*Clear cell ovarian cancer* originates in cells that line the uterus. Clear cell ovarian cancer is more like a kidney cancer in its molecular structure than other ovarian cancers, and the one that originates in the fallopian tube is actually like a particular breast cancer molecularly, i.e. in terms of the genes that are active and the way they behave.

This means anatomical classification of ovarian cancer is misleading. Knowledge about kidney cancer, in the case of the clear cell disease, and breast cancer, in the fallopian-tube-originating cancer, is more useful than knowledge about other ovarian cancers. This has brought about a big change in the way cancer is classified—it is beginning to be looked at in terms of the biology of the cancer, as opposed to its anatomy.

Professor Bowtell says there is no such 'single entity' any more as ovarian cancer or breast cancer—there are subtypes within subtypes, and the different types behave differently and need different treatment. 'The personalised medicine approach recognises that diversity, and tailors treatment to the particular subtype of disease an individual has,' he says. Ovarian cancer specialists now liaise with breast cancer specialists, and that type of cooperation happens across many separate cancer specialities.

The way some cancers are now being treated is completely different to how they were dealt with until recently. The professor says that the treatment of melanoma, for example, has been revolutionised by immunotherapy and targeted therapies that are prescribed on the principles of personalised medicine, and standard chemotherapy is now obsolete for melanoma.

Professor Bowtell explains that personalised medicine results in different approaches to treatment across different types of cancer: he says chemotherapy is still at the forefront of treating ovarian cancers, among others; approximately two-thirds of breast cancer treatments today are targeted therapies; and lung cancer treatment has been significantly impacted by immunotherapy and targeted therapies.

A targeted therapy means that doctors know what the particular mutation is in a patient and they give them a drug that targets that defect.

Platinum agents were developed in the 1970s and used as a standard chemotherapy treatment, and they appeared to successfully attack the DNA of some cancerous cells. The latest research has shown that they are actually a therapy that exploits a particular molecular defect, one found most commonly in a form of ovarian cancer. Because it is now known why they work and, more importantly which type of mutation they work on, they can be prescribed more effectively.

Arsenic targets a specific process that's disrupted in cells in a type of blood cancer called *acute promyelocytic leukaemia* (APL) and now, used in conjunction with a couple of other compounds in a targeted therapy, it has transformed survival rates for the condition. Previously APL was fatal for most people who developed it; now significant numbers of patients diagnosed with the condition are being cured.

## GETTING THE RIGHT THERAPY TO THE RIGHT PATIENT

As we have already seen in some of the examples cited by Professor Bowtell, personalised medicine has changed the way therapies are prescribed. In the US the FDA has approved more than a dozen drugs that target specific genetic mutations. They include imatinib—used to treat chronic myelogenous leukaemia—and the breast cancer drug trastuzumab.

As well as identifying which therapy might be most effective for an individual, a thorough understanding of genetics can also help doctors understand which drugs won't work for them. For example, if you are suffering from colon cancer and you have a genetic mutation called KRAS, there are two colon cancer drugs commonly used to treat this type of cancer that won't be prescribed as science has revealed that these therapies don't work when the KRAS mutation is involved.

Genetic profiling of a tumour is useful in helping doctors understand why another form of treatment, such as chemotherapy, hasn't been successful in the treatment of an individual. If they are able to identify a specific genetic mutation they may recommend a different drug, including those that that were originally designed to treat another type of cancer but have proved to be effective in the case of that patient's mutation.

◆ ◆ ◆

Personalised medicine is still in its infancy as a mainstream form of cancer treatment, but it has already helped us make huge strides in our understanding of how cancer develops, who is at risk of developing it, and how it might be treated.

Ongoing research is studying screening techniques that will enable doctors to identify the presence of cancer long before a patient develops the symptoms that normally prompt them to seek medical advice and be diagnosed with the condition.

The details it reveals about an individual's genetics will help doctors to prescribe the most appropriate therapy, which in turn will assist the pharmaceutical industry in developing ever-more-targeted therapies in the necessary volumes.

Although a 'new kid on the block', personalised medicine is—alongside immunotherapy—considered by researchers around the world as one of the most important developments in the history of the fight against cancer. Professor Peter Johnson, the chief clinician of Cancer Research UK, describes it as 'the most exciting change in cancer treatment since the invention of chemotherapy'. It is likely to revolutionise the diagnosis and treatment of not just cancer, but potentially a whole host of conditions that are related to our genetic make-up—Alzheimer's, diabetes and HIV AIDS among them.

# Chapter 9

# ELIMINATING ERROR CLINICAL TRIALS

The development of cancer treatments is cutting-edge science that requires a huge amount of testing at every stage. In this chapter we will:

◆ investigate the phases of development and clinical trials a new therapy must go through

◆ find out how patients can access cutting-edge therapies by getting onto a trial

◆ get the insights of a Research & Development expert at a major pharmaceutical company.

First, here's Jeremy's story of how chemotherapy gave him a second chance.

## 'Lazarus' rising

When James was first diagnosed with kidney cancer, he and his wife Sophie shared the reaction: 'This is one of those things life throws at you—we'll beat it, we'll get through.'

They spent hours every day researching the illness, quizzing their doctors and studying websites. A couple of months of investigation taught them that they had to temper their initial optimism. Everyone they spoke to and everything they read told them there was no cure for this form of cancer.

So James and Sophie steeled themselves for a long battle, and accepted the fact that the cancer was something James wasn't going to be able to get rid of. Their mindset was that they would make the most of the time they had left together.

Kidney cancer is generally resistant to chemotherapy and radiotherapy, so the doctors prescribed James a targeted therapy regime, intending to manage the condition and its symptoms. Despite the treatment James became weaker and they had to adapt their home accordingly. James lived on the ground floor when he reached a stage where he couldn't cope with the stairs.

Two and a half years after diagnosis James was only strong enough to take a few steps, and even speaking more than a few words at a time was beyond him. He was in a wheelchair the whole time he wasn't lying down, and scans showed the cancer was spreading aggressively through his lungs.

The therapy had not been able to hold the cancer, and the doctors told them James only had months to live. They went about the heartrending but necessary task of making sure all their affairs were in order and provisions made. Sophie's sister came to Sydney from her home in China to assist them in making funeral arrangements.

Sophie, however, was determined she would not leave one stone unturned in an attempt to stave off what now appeared to be the inevitable. She found out from their oncologist that the Westmead hospital in Sydney's western suburbs was conducting a trial into an immunotherapy drug for kidney cancer patients. The PD-1 antibody involved had proved successful in trials for melanoma and lung cancer patients, but this was the first time it was being tried out for patients like James.

One criterion for getting onto the trial involved James being able to achieve a far higher level of mobility than he had for a long time. For months he had not been able to walk anything like as far as he needed to in order to qualify—down the hospital corridor and into the consulting room of the specialist coordinating the trial. But he was determined to give it a go.

'I had to do it for my wife,' says James. 'Fundamentally I was too ill to be accepted onto the trial, but I just thought of her and put one foot in front of the other.' Putting mind over matter, James did enough to be accepted onto the trial, and started attending Westmead fortnightly for an infusion of the antibody. The treatment lasts two to three hours each visit.

Within one month of starting the trial James could walk twice as far as the 15 metres of corridor he had had to endure to get onto the trial. A month after that he was comfortably walking 100 metres, and four months after the first infusion he managed a kilometre. Nine months after starting on the PD-1 treatment James and Sophie went on a cruise—for 10 days, so he didn't miss his fortnightly appointment at the Westmead.

Today James still struggles with the stairs, and he can only take on gradual gradients on his walks, but says he has his 'life back'. Within weeks of incorporating a slight incline on his route to build up his stamina, he has progressed rapidly: from taking 15 minutes to walk a kilometre with a heart rate at completion of 128 bpm (beats per minute) to doing the same distance in nine minutes and finishing up at only 103 bpm. (Normal resting heart rate for adults is 60 to 100 bpm.)

James's latest scans reveal that half of his 'hot spots'—the areas of the body where the cancer is present—show reduced tumour sizes. The largest single one before treatment started, next to a rib, measured 80mm by 56mm—now it is 38mm by 26mm. One tumour has disappeared altogether. The remainder had increased slightly in size, but at a far slower rate than had been the case before James went onto the trial.

The only side effect James suffers as a result of the immunotherapy is a fever for a few hours when he gets home after each session.

He has found the support structure behind the trial a big step forward in managing all the treatment he requires. 'It makes such a difference having a clinical nurse to coordinate everything,' he says. 'When my saliva glands swelled up the nurse arranged for me to see the ear, nose and throat specialist, for example. Previously we would have had to sort all that out ourselves.'

James says the biggest thing he has learned from his experience is the importance of making certain you understand what is happening to you and what is going to happen to you. 'You have to keep asking the oncologist questions, and not be afraid to keep asking the same question until you really know what the answer means,' he says.

'And research, research, research!' If it wasn't for Sophie's work he wouldn't be on the trial, which he will be able to continue for as long as it produces positive results.

It is a sign of how far James has come that he now he feels tied to the hospital by an invisible cable, going in for treatment every two weeks. Initially the sessions were his entire focus, and it took all his strength to get in for them. Now he is doing so much more, and he and Sophie are able to travel interstate, but the length of any trip is governed by his fortnightly visits to Westfield.

'My clinical nurse calls me her Lazarus,' says James. 'When I started out my life expectancy was a matter of months. Two years later, despite still having the cancer, I can't believe how well I feel.'

No new drug can get the go-ahead from authorities to be released for public use without going through a clinical trial. Running a worthwhile drug trial relies on having enough of two fundamental resources— money and people. Constant publicity around the world emphasises the need to raise funds for cancer research, and most people would be aware of high-profile campaigns.

Once a new therapy has been designed, produced and tested in the laboratory, very careful assessment of its efficacy and side effects is needed. All therapies go through a series of clinical trials, starting with tiny sample groups in a highly-controlled environment. If the therapy passes this first phase of testing, further trials are conducted with larger groups of people. In the US, the FDA requires a therapy to go through four phases before licensing it:

◆ discovery and development

◆ preclinical research

◆ clinical research

◆ review.

Finding participants for trials does not receive the same level of publicity as funding, but is just as crucial.

Professor Robyn Ward is head of the Prince of Wales Clinical School and of the adult cancer program at the Lowy Cancer Research Centre, both located at the University of New South Wales in Sydney. Professor Ward emphasises that there is a lot of focus on securing donations from the public, which is very important, but that research needs people as well as dollars. Without large numbers of people volunteering to take part in clinical trials, many of the recent breakthroughs in cancer treatment would have taken years longer to achieve.

Professor Ward says, 'Many drugs for breast and bowel cancer that were trialled less than five years ago are now in routine care and we see patients benefit from them every day. Trials for new melanoma drugs have also had remarkable results.'

## COMPANY- VERSUS INVESTIGATOR-SPONSORED TRIALS

When a pharmaceutical company develops a drug and takes it into the clinic, the trial is described as *company sponsored*. Even when an investigator—a researcher or doctor, or group of researchers or doctors, at a particular hospital—says 'we're really interested in this trial and we'd like to be a site for it', the trial is still considered to be company sponsored because it has been initiated and set up by the drug company.

Sometimes, however, an investigator will say, 'We think this investigational treatment has potential opportunities that aren't being investigated—we think it's worth looking at what happens if you take drug X and combine it with drug Y in patient population Z.' The pharmaceutical company will consider the idea on its merits and may offer investigators the treatment at no cost so they can test it the way they envisage. In this case the trial is *investigator-sponsored*.

Similarly, doctors, or groups of doctors, at individual hospitals make breakthroughs themselves. They have an idea to create a drug to impact a specific molecule, or conceive a new way of carrying out a surgical procedure—the experimental work around these new ways of treating their patients is also described as investigator-sponsored trials. The key difference between company-sponsored and investigator-sponsored trials is where the concept behind the trial originally comes from.

## FROM CONCEPT TO CLINIC

When research indicates that a particular substance may be the basis for an effective treatment a rigorous process is followed, and it may take years for a treatment that is ultimately successful to make it onto the open market. For example, a therapeutic treatment that targets a specific protein called CTLA4 is now showing good results in the treatment of advanced melanoma. The idea of targeting the CTLA4 protein was originally conceived by Jim Allison in 1996—the FDA didn't actually license the first drug developed as a result of Allison's hypothesis, ipilimumab, until 2011.

### In vivo assays

Within all pharmaceutical companies the process for advancing a project into the clinic follows strict rules of governance. Animal experimentation is a controversial topic in many countries, but is an essential step for any drug before it moves into human clinical trials. Over time a great number of compounds were mooted as the potential basis for a drug that never even got as far as the clinic, because something absolutely critical was discovered during animal experimentation.

Researchers are open about imperfections in translating the science from an animal experiment to humans. No animals mirror exactly the behaviour in their cells—and reaction to changes in their cells—to those of humans. For this reason scientists do not refer to an 'animal model' but instead to an *in vivo assay*, meaning testing the effect a substance has on a living organism.

Dr Nils Lonberg, at time of writing Senior Vice President of Research & Development at Bristol-Myers Squibb, explains, 'The aim of these tests is to learn as much as possible about what is happening at a biological level in the interaction between the molecule we're putting into the in vivo assay and the readout that we get. To understand very well what the signal is and how that signal is interpreted is incredibly useful, and enables drugs to be selected to move on to human trials that have a higher likelihood of giving patient benefit without toxicity.'

All the drugs now available to the public are the product of a development process that uses well-understood and carefully-thought-out in vivo assays.

Following on from the premise that the cell biology of animals and humans is not identical, people may well ask the question: How do we know that things that don't work with in vivo assays won't work in humans? In other words, even if the drug didn't work—or had too harmful side effects—in the in vivo assays, that doesn't necessarily mean that it wouldn't work or would have the same effects on people.

Dr Lonberg at time of writing says this is a theory that is far too dangerous to put to the test, and that authorities would never countenance the initiation of human trialling purely on the back of untested theory. 'It would be a recipe for disaster to just rely on what a set of scientists think is a complete understanding of a biological system, without actually testing it as a biological system,' he says. 'There is too much that is not understood at this point in time about biology, and it would be arrogant to offer a drug to a human patient without first testing it in multiple ways.'

The in vivo assays are made on multiple species and usually take years to get to the stage where researchers and the authorities responsible for licensing drugs are comfortable that testing can begin on humans. In the case of a new drug, where the biology is well worked out and there is underlying science around the molecule behind it— such as when another drug has previously been devised and tested using a similar molecule—the drug can get into the clinic sooner. These are exceptional cases at the moment, and still take a year or more of pre-clinical work before human testing can begin.

### Steps towards licensing

Expectations are, however, that an increasing number of immunotherapy drugs will be able to be made available more quickly in the future. As more and more of these drugs are developed, and the knowledge base grows about their components, researchers and doctors will be able to get new drugs to a larger number of patients sooner. New products designed to behave in a slightly different way to those already on the market, but that are made up of the same compounds as existing drugs, can proceed to human trial sooner as the risks they pose are already known.

Once multiple tests have indicated that a drug will be safe to move into human trials it requires a licence from the relevant authority in the country in which it has been produced. The company has to prove to a health authority that, as Dr Lonberg explains, 'a medicine is what the company is saying that it is. We have to prove that it is free of contaminants and that we understand its effects.' Companies also have to show the authorities they can manufacture high volumes of the drug in a controlled way.

The next stage in the process for the company is to make a detailed case as to why their new drug should be taken further. They have to put together a scientific package to convince the regulatory authorities that the plan for testing the product is going to be worthwhile, and that it won't endanger the lives of patients.

They then approach institutional review boards at hospitals to persuade them, and their doctors, that their product has a good chance of being successful and will be suitable for the patients the hospital is treating at that time.

'The doctors themselves have to be convinced of the importance of the experiment to put their patients through the trial,' says Dr Lonberg, 'and they won't stage a trial unless they really think it will benefit their patients. Doctors are not there primarily to carry out experiments, they are there to treat and help people—yes, they do a lot of experiments, but only when they believe it may help their patients.

'It is important to have good science and a very compelling story before you even think about testing a medicine in the clinic,' Dr Lonberg adds.

Even then, there are occasions when a hospital will turn down a pharmaceutical company's request to run a trial despite the fact that they may believe the drug could be an important breakthrough. For example, if they don't see enough of a particular type of patient, and therefore aren't confident that they will be able to recruit enough people to conduct a worthwhile trial. Alternatively a hospital may already be running a trial, which they are very enthusiastic about, of another drug developed to impact on the same molecules, or a trial that is treating the same condition in another way.

## WHO TAKES PART IN TRIALS AND FOR HOW LONG?

Drug trials have strict eligibility criteria, to protect the participants and to optimise the quality of the results. However effective a new drug may potentially be to an ill patient, they need to be able to stand up to any side effects. The exhaustive testing done before a drug reaches the human trial stage informs doctors of particular groups of patients who would be at risk if exposed to a new drug, and unrelated health problems or symptoms that have arisen as a result of their disease will preclude some patients from being able to take part in trials.

The results of a trial are easier to interpret if the participants are clinically similar to each other. Drugs are usually aimed at patients whose cancer has reached the same stage of development, and the increasingly targeted nature of new therapies means that the selection criteria for trials are becoming narrower. As drugs now are often aimed at a specific mutation and individual proteins that are causing the cancer, more detail is required to find appropriate participants for trials—the upside is that, once identified, the targeted nature of the new drug means it is more likely to be effective for those patients.

Early-phase trials start out with small groups of participants, sometimes as few as 10 and rarely more than 100. Patients are initially given different doses of the drug being studied, to identify any side effects. This first phase can run for just a few months up to a year.

Adverse reactions to a new drug in the first phase of trialling don't necessarily mean that the whole concept has to be shelved. Sometimes the early phases of a clinical trial deliver encouraging results, but the drug causes unpleasant side effects. Previously the trial would have had to be discontinued and that drug discounted. Today, however, researchers do not have to go back to square one in these circumstances.

Advances in the identification of the elements that make up chemical and biological matter, and how they react to each other, mean the active ingredient in the drug may be usable in a different form or in a different dose. Researchers will mix the effective drug with other compounds in an effort to lessen the side effects, and look for other drugs with a similar chemical make-up that may not have the same side effects.

Once a drug has proved its safety it is measured against existing drugs in an expanded trial. Usually drugs will go through three or four phases of trials before they are licensed for public release, with more patients involved in each successive phase.

The second phase of a trial involves between 20 and a few hundred patients, and measures the effectiveness and ongoing safety for those receiving the drug over a couple of years. At this stage in the process a placebo is often introduced into a trial. A number of the participants are given completely inactive substances, against which the side effects and impact on the cancer experienced by those receiving the active new drug can be measured.

The third phase of a trial involves hundreds or even thousands of patients, and can be run simultaneously out of more than one hospital. During this phase the new drug is measured against a standard treatment already available for the same type of disease (if such a treatment exists), and usually lasts for at least two or three years.

A Phase IV trial is the continuous monitoring of a new drug once it has received a licence for widespread public use. It helps identify any side effects that arise from long-term use of a drug that are not evident in the early trial phases and monitors the effectiveness of the drug over time in a wider patient population.

Once all the phases of a trial are complete, support does not stop for the patients who have participated in them. James, who we met in the introduction to this section, will continue to receive his regular infusions of the PD-1 antibody at the hospital where the trial took place for as long as he derives benefit from it, irrespective of how long that is.

## HOW DO PATIENTS GET ONTO TRIALS?

The ongoing fight against all forms of cancer relies on the continued participation of large numbers of people in clinical trials. Anyone diagnosed with cancer potentially benefits themselves and fellow patients around the world by taking part in a clinical trial.

Dr Lonberg says patients are becoming increasingly sophisticated in researching upcoming trials and identifying those that they think may be appropriate for themselves. He believes they usually do this in discussion with their own doctors, although it is now possible, via the internet, for members of the public to find out the details of trials and how to get onto them—most of the public databases around the world include contact numbers of people coordinating each individual trial.

'I've met a lot of patients and I know a lot of patient stories,' says Dr Lonberg. 'It is very interesting the process that many of them went through to get onto a particular trial. In many cases it was their doctor who recommended a clinical trial, but in many other cases the patient was very active, doing a lot of their own research to find a suitable trial.'

Pharmaceutical companies also field enquiries from patients and doctors when they hear about drugs that a company is developing. In these cases the companies can act as intermediaries, to put the patient's doctor in touch with those investigators conducting trials.

'We as a company cannot decide what is appropriate for a patient,' says Dr Lonberg. 'It is the patient's treating doctor and the doctors conducting the trial who decide whether or not a trial is right for specific patients.' He emphasises that the relationship between a doctor and a patient determines what form treatment takes, and drug companies are never involved in the decision-making process for individuals.

## HARNESSING ADVANCED TECHNOLOGIES IN TRIALS

Advanced technologies, including artificial intelligence (AI), are now helping research teams address the most challenging aspects of drug development. Regulations and standards in clinical research are becoming ever more complex, adding to the time and cost of getting therapies to market. Pharmaceutical companies are using AI to improve the efficiency of clinical trials and to identify and enrol patients onto them.

AI allows researchers to create algorithms that help identify potential molecular targets for new drugs far more quickly than was previously possible. Predictive models are being used to assess their potential success before going to the effort and expense of commencing development of the drugs themselves.

The conception and development of a new therapy involves an enormous amount of data, and AI and automation enable information to be processed and analysed far more quickly. Because AI is in its infancy and developing rapidly, the medical science community sees huge potential for its contribution to the quicker development of new therapies in years to come.

## MORE TRIALS MEAN BETTER RESULTS

The first checkpoint inhibitor immunotherapy was approved by the FDA in 2011, and adoptive cell therapy was first used to treat a leukaemia patient in 2012. Since then, more and more immunotherapies have been released onto the market every year. That acceleration is a result of research that has been going on for many years, with a marked increase in activity in this area since the early 2000s.

The whole body of work behind immunotherapy is like an iceberg, and the late clinical work is the tip of the iceberg when trials bring it into public consciousness.

'There has been a decade of fundamental science and drug discovery around a lot of different pathways for immuno-oncology,' says Dr Lonberg. 'The results of the work are becoming apparent at a rapid rate, but that doesn't mean it's just happening now.'

He also stresses the importance of the backing of the wider medical community in the increase in the number of products becoming available to patients.

'There is a very large number of trials ongoing,' he says, 'and that is a reflection of the enthusiasm of the major medical centres and the physicians at the major medical centres. That in turn is driven by the data. It is the underlying science that is behind the increase in the new generation of drugs that patients are now getting access to.'

Most countries around the world have public databases that enable residents to find out about all the trials taking place in that country, what the criteria are for being accepted into trials, and how to apply to become involved in them. Doctors are being encouraged to be aware of trials taking place in their particular field so they can discuss trials with their patients, and give more details about trials to help their patients to make a well-informed decision about taking part.

◆ ◆ ◆

Trials still tend to run below full capacity around the world, so there is scope for more patients to reap the benefits of taking part in clinical trials. Being involved in a clinical trial potentially improves the chances of making a recovery, or managing cancer with a better quality of life, and contributes to the body of knowledge that will help to fight the disease in all its forms globally. A collective effort is needed by governments, healthcare providers and patients to ensure every clinical trial involves as many people as it is designed to accommodate.

## Chapter 10

# THE HUMAN ELEMENT PSYCHOSOCIAL ONCOLOGY

Psychosocial oncology has emerged as the missing link in cancer care—one that focuses on the whole person, rather than the medical aspects of treatment alone.

The term psychosocial oncology is made up of three parts:

◆ psycho—relating to the mind or the psyche

◆ social—concerned with the relationships people have with family and with society

◆ oncology—meaning the branch of medicine that deals with cancer.

In other words, psychosocial oncology is a speciality in cancer care concerned with understanding and treating the social, psychological, emotional, spiritual, quality-of-life and functional aspects of cancer, from diagnosis, treatment, survivorship, palliative care and prevention through to bereavement.

To start with, Bruce's ongoing journey.

## Living with melanoma

In early 2009, Bruce was a fit and healthy 55-year-old large-animal veterinarian who had played A-grade cricket until he was 46. During a routine visit to a medical clinic, he mentioned a lump on the top of his head. 'Don't worry,' the doctor said, 'it's only an infected pimple.' Over the following months, Bruce knocked the lump a few times; it bled and never healed.

Six months later he knew he was in trouble. 'I was having a shower and my neck was sore; moving my head around I felt a huge lump, 4cm x 2.5cm, under my collarbone. That was when my vet skills said, Oh-oh, that is in a regional lymph node; we've got a problem.'

This new lump under his collarbone was probably secondary to the primary lesion at the back of his scalp.

A new GP examined it. 'Why did you wait so long to come and see me about this?' he exclaimed. Bruce probably had cancer, he said, 'but don't let's get ahead of ourselves'. He sent off samples that came back positive, and referred Bruce to Melbourne's Peter MacCallum Cancer Centre (Peter Mac).

'Biopsies of the lump on my scalp and the lump tucked in behind my right collarbone confirmed that I had metastatic melanoma,' Bruce recalls. 'But at Peter Mac, they were doing all sorts of tests over a few weeks, to work out where the cancer had spread and whether I was a Stage 3 or a Stage 4 patient. This was critical regarding my surgery and also important regarding my prognosis. There was a lump inside my right pelvis—in the psoas muscle—that glowed with PET scan dye. There was also a shadow in my right lung on X-ray.'

Bruce was at Peter Mac on visit three or four when a passing doctor noticed his cheerfulness. He checked his file and asked, 'Has anyone told you that with this type of cancer 50% of people are dead within five years?'

No one had: 'I just went white.' Then Bruce collected his thoughts. 'Please don't misunderstand me when I say that I'm really sorry about the 50% who are going to die. But I'm going to be one of the 50% who live.'

'Yep, fair enough,' the doctor said. He just wanted to give Bruce a reality check.

Bruce knows now he was at Stage 3B, meaning the cancer had spread into nearby tissues or lymph nodes and was about to spread into other areas of the body. He became 'case of the month' as Peter Mac searched worldwide for similar patients.

It took a month to be seen by specialists. 'A month seemed like an eternity… every day was challenging for me.' The cancer had spread so fast that Bruce was anxious to catch it before it spread further. His GP understood, but no one else realised how much the uncertainty knocked him around mentally, triggering both anxiety and frustration that they couldn't do something ASAP.

Having lived alone since 1992, Bruce didn't deal with his anxiety 'textbook style'. He would be able to put on his 'veterinarian hat' when he had a better idea of how the cancer would behave.

Now a division opened up between doctors—the 'sarcoma' team wanted to hop in early, operate and get out the lump in his pelvis quickly before it caused any more problems, whereas the 'melanoma' team said, 'Whoa, we need to do a bit more homework here before we rush in.' The problem with surgery was that the psoas muscle holds the top of the femur into the pelvis, so cutting that out would mean Bruce would have an unstable leg, walk with a limp, and be in chronic pain for the rest of his life.

The two competing sections considered a biopsy of this glowing lesion, but going in with a long biopsy needle raised risks of contamination and bowel perforation.

St Vincent's looked at the scans and said they could do it, so Bruce went in with an overnight bag. However, when they did their own scan they said, 'Sorry, you're too high-risk; we're not going to do a biopsy now.' The uncertainty continued—a chest X-ray showed shadows on the lungs, indicating metastasis. Yet that turned out to be a false alarm.

Extensive surgery of his head, neck and shoulder was scheduled in early September 2009.

His ex-wife, Pam, was the first person Bruce rang. 'Have you told the kids yet?' she asked. He hadn't, so she rang their grown-up daughter and son and arranged dinner to break the news.

This diagnosis was bigger than anything Bruce had fought before and he would not be able to do it by himself. He was going to need somewhere to stay to recuperate post-surgery. His father had died in 1988 and his elderly mother made it clear early on that he couldn't stay at her house. His two-years-younger sister Sally said no; so did his brother Don.

Bruce felt devastated. It was hard to ask for help, even harder to accept rejection.

Finally, his PhD supervisor in Beechworth gained two weeks compassionate leave to look after him. 'I will be forever in debt to her—she was there when my own family abandoned me.'

Friends drove down from Wodonga to pick up him up after the surgery, but a problem with sutures meant they had to drive back without him. Another family came down later to pick him up.

Bruce got the all-clear at the three-month review in December. Then 10 days later, Sally was diagnosed with ovarian cancer. 'They got her health up to par so they could open her up then they said, "No, sorry. There is nothing that we can do for you," and sewed her back together again.'

That hit Bruce hard. 'Suddenly the boot was on the other foot. I realised how helpless I was when it was someone else who got the diagnosis of cancer.'

Two years later, before Sally died, she said, 'I'm going to die, you're going to survive; it's up to you to give back to the cancer community.' He promised that he would do his best.

In January 2010, Bruce had to decide whether to have radiation therapy. 'I put on my vet hat: without radiotherapy it had a 66%

chance of not coming back; with radiotherapy that was boosted to 87%.'

That was not a big jump once side effects were considered, so Bruce declined the offer. His daughter was 21 and his son just turning 18, so 'just in case I did die', he decided on overseas travel for six weeks with them instead. 'Six weeks to find out how your children tick was just brilliant.'

In December 2010 Bruce was returning from another trip and felt a lump the size of a large pea in the parotid region under his right ear. He drove straight to Peter Mac and the melanoma was operated on within a month.

Once the scars were healed they said, 'You don't have a choice this time; you need radiation therapy.' Bruce had to come to Melbourne for the 23 days of radiotherapy; the hospital accommodation was being refurbished so organising accommodation was 'a nightmare'.

Bruce had moved to Leongatha in regional Victoria for a career change in his government vet job, but a new boss bullied him into a mental breakdown in mid-2011. He ceased work and returned to Melbourne in 2014.

But Bruce's cancer journey didn't end there. The melanoma can sit there dormant for five, 10, 20 years and then flare up when the immune system weakens. 'Pretty much every year I had a new lump, a new investigation. Anyone with a diagnosis of cancer gets anxious about new lumps. They even have a name for it—scan-anxiety—getting it examined may be stressful in itself.'

After this happening yearly for three or four years, family and friends got sick of the uncertainty: 'Have you got cancer, or haven't you?' After a while Bruce gave up sharing where he was up to.

'It's a complicated twist to the cancer journey that sometimes the only person you can go to is a professional,' he says. 'I didn't have a close partner to share it with. I knew I mustn't burden my children—

it was hard enough for them to see me sick. I met a wonderful counsellor named Amanda after my workplace-bullying incident and she's guided me for eight years.'

The lump that was glowing in the psoas muscle continued to be a mystery. Today, specialists think it's a benign tumour called a *neurofibroma*.

In remission, Bruce stays fit, eats healthy. 'In the early part after the diagnosis, I kept a diary about how I was feeling—that was a good tool. To think about it enough to put it into words helps me to get it into perspective. I have a host of longstanding pain issues and the only way I could answer honestly whether I have any pain was to wean myself off the doses of painkillers. It helped the doctors to measure how the cancer was behaving in my body; it was useful dealing with side effects of my radiation therapy; we could easily map any changes. That was a coping mechanism that worked for me.'

Bruce now volunteers his time to help other people along their cancer journey. As a vet with his own private practice he understands clinical process, and his own long journey gives him first-hand experience and knowledge. He is involved with three melanoma support groups and a head-and-neck-cancer patient support group.

'You get back manyfold what you give,' Bruce says. 'Cancer can just stay hidden and waiting inside a person's body—there is so much we do not know. If the cancer does come back, I hope I have learned coping strategies that I can share with these groups. I'm not fatalistic; I'm realistic.'

He is a member of the psychosocial committee under the Peter Mac board, which meets monthly, and the Wellness Centre contacts him for help with other projects.

He remembers feeling overwhelmed by the hustle and bustle the first time he walked in to Peter Mac. 'Cancer care has come a long way since 2009.' He was appointed a case manager who took a lot of the worry out of organising test results—a senior nurse who looked after 20 patients.

But there was no case manager when the cancer came back in December 2010 and his experience was 'horrendous', with staff not ready for appointments and no accommodation available during radiation therapy.

We were saddened to learn in August 2021 that Bruce had been diagnosed with prostate cancer. 'Apparently there is a link between these cancers,' he comments. 'I didn't know that previously. A timely warning for men with these cancers.'

This time round, his two adult children are there to support him.

Prostate-removal surgery in late September went well, but they discovered a whole new cancer: a diffuse large B-cell lymphoma, which is an aggressive type of non-Hodgkin lymphoma that develops from the B-cells in the lymphatic system.

'We have caught it early so my chances of survival should be pretty good,' he says.

Cancer isn't going away anytime soon. Advances in treatment mean many more survivors, making survivorship a hot topic. Bruce has been working with Peter Mac on its hospital patient-discharge policy, so once people leave the supportive hospital environment and return home to the reality of everyday life, they have help and support at their fingertips.

'After being lucky enough to still be in remission, it's just my way of saying thank you to the doctors and all the wonderful people who've kept me alive,' Bruce says. And he is still keeping his promise to Sally.

Psychosocial oncology has emerged as the missing link in cancer care—one that focuses on the whole person, rather than the medical aspects of treatment alone.

The cancer journey can be one of the toughest that a person will ever have to travel. As we have seen with Bruce's story, a plethora of human needs will come up during each stage of the disease, not only for that person, but for those around them.

Psychosocial oncology, also known as psycho oncology, aims to improve the quality of life for everyone involved. It's a speciality in cancer care concerned with understanding and treating the six aspects of cancer:

◆ social

◆ psychological

◆ emotional

◆ spiritual

◆ quality of life

◆ functional.

Research shows that psychosocial oncology works. In randomised controlled trials, people with cancer receiving psychological therapies showed improvements of 10–14% in adjusting emotionally, functioning socially, managing treatment- and disease-related symptoms, and improved quality of life. And people with cancer who received psycho-educational or psychosocial interventions showed much lower rates of anxiety, depression, mood disorders, nausea, vomiting and pain. They also had greater knowledge about the disease and its treatments.

Professor Steve Ellen is Director of the Psychosocial Oncology Program at Peter MacCallum Cancer Centre. As a teaching and practising psychiatrist, he has 20 years' experience in the emergency department of The Alfred Hospital.

'When you talk about cancer,' Dr Ellen explains, 'most people focus on the medical aspects—the surgery, the physicians, the medications, the oncologists and the radiation therapy—and the side effects and how it all goes. And that gets all the attention.

'And one thing that's come about, more or less in the last 15 years, is the realisation that while we're making some great advances in the medical side of cancer, we've probably left the rest behind a little bit.'

## AN EMOTIONAL ROLLER-COASTER

A person with cancer may ride an emotional roller-coaster, with feelings ranging from anger or sadness to fear or helplessness. People may feel they no longer have any control over their situation, or perhaps their feelings are so mixed that they are hard to separate. These feelings often come and go—the good news is that they usually improve with time as the person gets used to their diagnosis and treatment, and learns how to handle the stress of having cancer.

Essentially, Dr Ellen says, psychosocial oncology is concerned with 'how the person is coping with their illness'. This includes everything from the mental illnesses they might get, to the psychological adjustments they have to make, to specific issues they need to deal with.

Mental illnesses such as depression and anxiety are 'quite common' in cancer.

'About one-quarter of people get depression or anxiety, depending on the cancer,' Dr Ellen says. 'Anxiety is very common in cancer, especially around the treatments—people often get anxiety leading into treatments and before each round of chemotherapy.'

People also need to get used to all the changes that are happening. 'There's all the psychological aspects,' Dr Ellen explains, 'not so much mental illness but there's adjusting, for example to disfiguring surgery; you might have to have surgery on your face, or your breasts removed and reconstructed.'

For someone to adapt to these kinds of surgeries, they need to pass through various stages of grief. 'Grieving is a process and some people don't go through it very well and so they might get stuck at a particular point and find they just can't move on,' Dr Ellen says.

However, not everyone experiences grief in a linear set of stages. The five common stages of grief experienced by terminally ill patients that Elisabeth Kübler-Ross discussed in her 1969 classic *On Death and Dying*—denial and isolation; anger; bargaining; depression; acceptance—have been found to be only a guide. People who are grieving do not necessarily go through the stages in the same order, or experience all of them. Or sometimes they can get stuck and find it hard to move through a stage.

## CHALLENGES ACROSS THE SPECTRUM

Problems may also come up in managing all the various family relationships. 'There's lots of specific issues,' Dr Ellen says. 'For example, how do you be a parent when you've got cancer? How do you find time? What do you tell your kids, how do you explain it?'

So psychosocial oncology deals with a diverse set of challenges that range right across the spectrum from the emotional and the psychological to the physical and the practical.

These may begin with coping with the shock of diagnosis, and a person fearing for their health and their future.

Physical symptoms and adverse effects of treatment may include nausea, fatigue, sleep problems, and changes in body appearance and physical functioning.

In practical terms, financial costs, altered work and financial status can cause trouble.

Psychological difficulties range from concerns about body image and sexuality to disorders such as anxiety and/or depression. Some people will have to face the prospect of progressive illness and impending death.

This huge range of non-medical issues requires a team made up of many disciplines:

◆ clinical psychologists

◆ social workers

- psychiatrists and psychiatric registrars

- consultation—liaison nurses.

## A TEAM APPROACH

Dr Ellen's team at the psychosocial oncology program combines psychological, psychiatric and social into one area, using effective, evidence-based treatments.

People bring in questions to do with many issues:

- adjusting to having cancer

- accepting body changes

- managing relationships

- fearing the cancer coming back

- relaxing or sleeping better

- managing depression and anxiety

- making treatment decisions.

The clinical psychology team offers psychological therapies and interventions—from cognitive behaviour therapy to mindfulness, acceptance and commitment therapy, and existential psychotherapy—tailoring it to people's needs.

The psychiatric team aims to improve mental health by assessing and planning treatment for people with both cancer and mental health problems. The treatments may include psychological, pharmacological and social approaches.

Counselling can help with planning for the future, bereavement, legal and financial support, community resources and advance care planning.

Music therapy is an internationally practised, evidence-based profession that may help with reducing experiences of pain, breathlessness, sleeplessness or anxiety, whether listening to recorded music, making music or experiencing music played by the therapist. It's also pleasurable 'time out' while in hospital.

Dr Ellen works closely with the Director of Prevention & Wellbeing, Geraldine McDonald, who oversees a modern, elegant wellbeing centre. Together, they aim to design a seamless experience to ensure the patient is given the best care across the different departments.

## A TAILORED APPROACH

Triage is crucial to this new collaborative approach, so that people are allocated the best care for their individual situation. This treatment is driven by their individual needs, rather than taking a hospital-driven, one-size-fits-all approach.

This is a radical change from the old, paternalistic system where the doctor was a godlike figure who expected unquestioning compliance with the course of treatment from both staff and patient.

Patient-centred care involves another consideration in planning, delivering and evaluating services, adds Dr Ellen—staying within the patient's belief system, whether spiritual, religious or cultural.

The team members assess patients who are at risk of mental health problems within the framework of their cancer journey, whether the problems are pre-existing or current.

Diagnosis is made up of four stages:

◆ ask questions to diagnose

◆ recommend treatment and explain options

◆ seek patient agreement (informed consent)

◆ encourage questions.

### Measuring effectiveness

Gaining funding for a psychosocial oncology department wasn't as straightforward as putting up a strong case for funding more recognisable medical treatment, where the numbers such as survival or speed of recovery are easily measurable. It's harder to convince funding bodies when it comes to psychosocial benefits. How do you measure quality of life? What kinds of key performance indicators could you use for something like wellbeing, which seems so intangible?

But 'solid evidence' is there, Dr Ellen says, which shows that looking after the psychosocial aspects of patients suffering cancer results in a drop in the length of hospital stays. In addition, people manage their treatment better—taking medications and showing up for appointments and treatments—resulting in quicker recovery. Research also shows the treatment of emotional problems—including anxiety and depression—results in fewer visits to both GPs and specialists, giving big savings in medical billing.

## RECOGNISING AND RESPONDING TO NEEDS

It's only recently that mental illnesses such as depression have been publicly recognised as being widespread in the community.

'We're responding to mental illness better now and beyondblue has helped bring it into national awareness,' Dr Ellen says. And with prominent sportspeople and celebrities acknowledging their own personal struggles, our society has become much more open about our vulnerability.

It's been found that 35–47% of cancer patients experience significant psychological distress, more often when there's a greater risk of death. When people need to be hospitalised for a diagnosis, treatment or palliative care, losing their involvement in their various family, work or leisure roles can compound their distress.

Symptoms of distress include trouble sleeping, feeling hungry, concentrating and, in general, carrying on with daily life. However, only 5% seek psychological help. This affects how they cope with their illness as well as how they adhere to their treatment regime.

Coping with a life-threatening illness can be sufficiently horrifying and intense to have the potential to lead to post-traumatic stress disorder (PTSD); those who have been diagnosed and treated for cancer at a young age are vulnerable to trauma from aspects like painful procedures and frightening separation from their parents.

A cancer diagnosis has added potential to amplify or bring back PTSD from past experiences. Monash University's Professor Paul Mullen initially recognised that trauma and PTSD are not restricted to soldiers in a war zone. In a ground-breaking study in the 1990s, he showed that they can result from childhood, from domestic and sexual violence.

For busy hospital staff, it's easy to see that the most visibly affected people need help, but the others may be left to go downhill until they are obviously in a bad way—many are reluctant to report their feelings of distress to healthcare providers.

So that staff could quickly identify at-risk people, Peter Mac introduced in early 2016 a mandatory distress screening at the point of entry to specialist clinics. The tool is called the Distress Thermometer and Problem Checklist. This measures distress on a scale of zero to 10, where 10 is the worst, similar to the more common way of measuring pain.

When this tool was used in an acute haematology and oncology ward of Melbourne's The Alfred hospital in 2006, 51% of patients were identified as being significantly distressed, of whom 47% had not received psychosocial support before screening. A substantially higher number of emotional and physical problems was reported by significantly distressed patients. During this pilot study, referrals to psychology and social work services increased. Once screening was directing more patients into care, it helped staff care for their patients better and most agreed that some form of routine screening should continue.

## PSYCHOSOCIAL SURVIVORSHIP

The number of cancer survivors has swelled steadily over the past decades. Most cancer survivors have been found to cope well with the after-effects of their illness.

However, surviving doesn't necessarily mean a life free of problems, whether related to the disease or after-effects of treatment—they may include pain, fatigue, psychological distress and struggling to participate in work.

Psychosocial survivorship supports people as they move beyond their treatment and adjust to life after cancer.

A traumatic event such as being diagnosed for cancer can help us grow stronger. We can respond to adversity in four ways:

◆ by succumbing to it

◆ by surviving with a poorer quality of life

◆ by returning to our original quality of life, or

◆ by thriving—that is, finding meaning and creativity in the experience.

That's where psychosocial oncology can really come into its own.

Chapter 11

# LIVING WITH CANCER

For someone living with cancer, staying as strong as possible is vital to help fight the disease. Maintaining resilience and energy levels will help the body cope with treatment and improve the chances of that treatment being successful, as well as bolstering the immune system.

A robust body and mind and an effective immune system can also help to prevent cancer recurring in the future.

In this chapter we will reveal:

◆ the best approach to nutrition, exercise and sleep

◆ the complementary therapies that supplement treatment

◆ how to go about helping someone with cancer

◆ improving quality of life with palliative care

◆ some secrets to survivorship.

Alexandra's inspiring story shows how it's possible to emerge stronger after a cancer ordeal.

## A recipe for resilience

Alexandra (Alyx to her friends) Stewart used to work as an orthoptist in several ophthalmology practices as well as studying forensic science in her 'non-existent' spare time.

After Alyx found a tiny lump in her right breast, she mentioned it to a doctor—not her regular GP—during a Pap smear. The doctor could not feel the lump: 'It's probably just hormonal. Besides, you're too young to have breast cancer.'

Almost 18 months later, Alyx and her fiancé were planning their wedding when the lump seemed to grow overnight, and became painful. She visited her regular GP for tests and the results indicated she needed to have a mastectomy.

'When I fronted up to the surgeon's office for the first time, he couldn't understand a word I was saying through the tears,' she says. 'It was nine weeks to walking down the aisle in my dream dress and I would look like a freak.'

Alyx was soon to turn 36. She felt strongly that a postponed wedding would never go ahead in the future... if there was a future.

She was unprepared for the pain after her first mastectomy, and the experience was made worse by not having a breast-care nurse to prepare her for surgery.

'I couldn't draw in a decent breath for a couple of weeks and I couldn't stop shaking from shock,' she recalls. 'I wondered why the truck that had clearly run over me in the operating theatre had not finished off the job.'

The chemotherapy started, and again it was 'horrendous'—the hospital tried in vain to stop the continuous vomiting. Alyx was admitted for a few days after each session to deal with the nausea.

Alyx made it down the aisle, but they couldn't go on their white Christmas honeymoon to Canada. They each wept on their wedding night.

Many surgeries followed, and some 'not so brilliant' hospital stays. 'My husband was almost a widower after four months of marriage.'

The signs were pointing to a future breast cancer diagnosis, and Alyx opted to have her other breast removed.

'In the end, skin-saving mastectomies with implants have been exactly right for me,' she says.

Alyx didn't cope well through any of her treatment, and chose to shun the world, her friends and most of her family.

She eventually returned to work, even managing to finish that forensic science degree. 'But I was changed. Life was beginning to expect more from me.' When elderly patients said to her, 'Don't get old', they didn't realise that not getting old was her biggest fear, and a privilege many of her friends would not have.

Cancer taught Alyx a lesson: how to learn to survive happily.

'Survivorship is my greatest challenge,' she says. 'Thoughts of cancer and recurrence can lie dormant—it can take only one ill-thought statement from someone and I am right back there in cancer headspace.'

Counselling was valuable for her obsessive-compulsive disorder and panic attacks.

'I had to look for a way through,' she says. 'That's when I came across this technique. If I could find one positive in my life, no matter how small, and work with that, I might be able to get through each day. I started with how lucky I was to have a gorgeous cat.

'I would place pictures on a board of really simple things I liked, and I built on those.'

Once Alyx was making vision boards, she was admitting that she had a future—she could now dream of the things she was going to do.

'At times, survivor's guilt still crops up,' she says. 'I give it the space it needs and let the emotions flow. Then I get on with the living part.'

Alyx's horrendous journey had led her to see that many people have similar experiences and frustrations while going through cancer treatment.

'How can I help these people?' she asked herself.

Her biggest frustration had been the lack of communication between herself and those around her.

'I needed help, they wanted to help and yet the two rarely came together,' she says. 'Asking for help is intimidating. Friends and family of cancer patients often do all the things you don't need.'

There had to be a better way. In 2014 she launched iCare4u, an app for cancer sufferers. It rallies friends and family in the virtual world so they can help in the real world, keeping everyone connected and communicating. The sufferer, or someone they trust, lists the tasks that need doing and the helpers assign themselves to a task.

She enjoys the feedback from app users, knowing she has made a positive impact for someone else.

'My proudest moment was having iCare4u featured on Channel 9's *Today* show,' Alyx says.

In the meantime, Alyx's parents had travelled their own cancer journey—her mother survived, but not her father. And like Alyx and many others, he struggled with food intake, eating very little. For months Alyx had got by on a severely restricted diet when she could eat only 'lamb, garlic, the freshest white bread and jam', losing 10kg.

Adding cancer side effects to inadequate nutrition leaves the body rundown and 'less able to fight a good fight', potentially leading to malnutrition. In fact, she found that up to 80% of people become malnourished during their cancer treatment.

So Alyx enlisted the help of a dietitian to develop Kee-moh Snacks, a range of nutritious foods packed with protein, amino acids and clean ingredients. Each product contains lists of side effects it is suited to, for the days people don't feel like eating.

Kee-moh Snacks has now grown to become Centre For Cancer Nutrition—the go-to hub for everything cancer-nutrition-related. Its quarterly magazine focuses on using seasonal produce for maximum flavour and freshness, with recipes suggesting adaptations to make them suitable for various treatment side effects. Alyx has certainly found her calling.

She finds it rewarding to reassure and inform others by speaking about her experience as a Breast Cancer Network Australia volunteer community liaison.

While training for that role, she met a breast cancer dragon boater. Paddling dragon boats for breast cancer had begun in Canada in 1996 to disprove the theory that strenuous upper-body exercise after mastectomy brings on lymphoedema. Alyx went along to give it a go. 'Before I knew it, I was a signed-up member. Soon after, my husband joined too.'

Dragon boating has taken the couple around the country and overseas for competitions. Water sport, like public speaking and television appearances, is something Alyx would never have done prior to cancer.

'I love my work,' Alyx says. 'It is far more interesting than it might have turned out, had it not been for cancer.'

---

The three pillars of health are even more essential for people living with cancer:

◆ eating the right things consistently

◆ maintaining some form of regular exercise

◆ getting enough sleep.

These three pillars complement each other—doing one makes it easier to do the others—and helps both mental and physical wellbeing.

We have seen throughout this book how an integrated approach to cancer treatment increases its success; in the same way, people with cancer can improve both their chances of survival and their quality of life by being as healthy in mind—including having a positive attitude to coping with, and fighting, cancer—and body as possible.

## EATING WELL

Eating well is crucial to maintaining strength, but people with cancer often find it difficult to motivate themselves to eat.

For most—and this was confirmed by everyone we spoke to for the patient stories in this book—the mental side of cancer is the hardest thing to deal with. Some say that the physical discomfort from the side effects of treatment saps their motivation, often becoming more dispiriting than the pain of the disease itself. Staying motivated is even harder when they feel weak, so they have to overcome this lack of motivation to avoid going into a downward spiral of lethargy and weakness.

Most of our interviewees make sure to not use hunger or a desire to eat as a trigger. They keep their strength up by eating at the same times each day, and eat small amounts more often as they do not feel like big meals.

Many hospitals have dietitians who see patients regularly throughout treatment, guiding them on symptom management and also managing their diet to maintain weight and a good nutritional status—that is, preventing and managing malnutrition, as well as managing weight loss during treatment if they've got side effects and are not eating.

Dietitians tailor their support according to needs—some people need individualised diets and others need just some general information.

For a while people may be eating lots of higher-protein, higher-calorie foods just to try and maintain their energy intake, because there can be a much higher requirement for energy and protein during treatment.

Following treatment, the priority is to get back to a good or a stable weight, and then transition to more of a normal diet.

## Fortifying foods

It's important to make everything count towards regenerating the body. 'You may need to get a full day's nutrition into the one morsel you're able to get down that day,' Alyx Stewart says.

The key here is to go further than selecting the best foods and think in terms of fortifying them as well, so that each mouthful is a nutrient powerhouse.

A good way to fortify food is to start with a base such as fruit, soup or vegetables and add extra things such as oils, butter, cream or cheese to get the most out of the small amounts a person with cancer may be able to eat.

Peanut butter is nutritious and easy on the mouth if you select the smooth variety. You can also stir it into porridge. It goes well with sweet chilli sauce, strong cheddar and green beans.

For a smoothie, you can select a milk and then add all sorts of other things. Soy milk offers a good alternative to cow's milk, especially for vegans—it is always fortified with calcium and has good protein content. Almond milk is not as rich in protein. Many 'milks' end up being fortified with calcium, but it's important to check the quantities on the labels because they may differ nutritionally from cow's milk.

Next, add fruit and then ice cream, yoghurt and/or a protein powder. (In terms of a brand of protein powder, dietitians will suggest one depending on the person's nutritional needs.)

The benefit of making dairy a key component of a smoothie is that it will have protein, fats and other nutrients as well as some dairy sugars. Every mouthful will offer up the most nutritious combination of nutrients, rather than filling up on empty calories.

According to Vasanti Malik, a nutrition research scientist at the Harvard TH Chan School of Public Health, US: 'Dairy isn't necessary in the diet for optimal health, but for many people, it is the easiest way to get the calcium, vitamin D, and protein they need to keep their heart, muscles and bones healthy and functioning properly.'

For a single go-to dairy source, Malik recommends plain Greek yoghurt. (Flavoured versions are high in sugar.) 'It has more protein than regular yoghurt and contains probiotics that help with gut health,' she says. 'You can eat it alone or add it to other dishes like smoothies and use it as a substitute for cream in recipes.'

Soups offer endless nourishing options, particularly if someone is finding it hard to swallow, and especially if they have added protein such as minced meat, fish or legumes. Meat can be blended in if it is too hard to swallow. Lentils can be added to make a chunky soup rather than a broth; there's not a lot of nutritional value in a broth. (See Chapter 12 for 1001 ways with a can of soup.)

### *Protein is crucial*

Your body needs protein to build and repair tissues, and turns it over constantly. Normally it breaks down the same amount of protein that it uses for its building and repair work. However, at other times— typically in periods of illness—it breaks down more protein than it can create, thus increasing your body's needs.

Australian grass-fed protein is one of the best in the world. Whey protein from milk is also valuable, flavoured with clean cacao or organic vanilla, and sweetened with stevia or monk-fruit powder (which is sweeter than stevia) rather than sugar.

When you start with fruit you can fortify it with some protein by adding things like yoghurt, ice cream or custard.

For a vegan, the most problematic thing may be getting enough protein to build up strength, as well as replenish what has been lost. For vegetarians, this is less difficult as they have high-protein dairy options such as cow's milk for both food and drink.

Vegans can use foods like soy milk and soy products as well as nuts and tofu; legumes are high in protein, particularly soybeans, chickpeas, lentils, and peanuts. Quinoa is a superfood that's high in protein as well as vitamins, minerals and fibre. Many vegetarian alternatives are also vegan appropriate, using an almond or a soy milk as the best choice for smoothies. Because coconut yoghurt and coconut products are not high in protein, they are not recommended as a suitable alternative to the other milk types.

## The skinny on fats

Although it isn't helpful to be overweight, weight loss is common among people with all forms of cancer, and is often a consequence of treatment.

Protein, fats and carbohydrates are an important part of the diet for those who are underweight. Cancer patients should not shy away from foodstuffs containing them, because it is important to get a balanced diet from all these nutrients.

However, some people may struggle to eat a balanced diet due to feeling unwell. A dietitian will support them to build up their diet focusing on higher energy foods, such as adding fats (avocado, olive oil, cheese, cream, butter) and protein (dairy, nuts, eggs, fish) to help prevent further weight loss. A tablespoonful of cream added to pumpkin soup will make it creamier and add some calories in the form of fat, or a beaten egg can be stirred into soup just before serving.

'If it needs to be high fat, then make it high fat,' Alyx Stewart says.

Coconut products are rich in fats, which can give energy, but the fat is saturated, meaning it is not as healthy for your body. For the general healthy population, dietitians tend to suggest not overdoing the coconut products because most people who are well don't need the extra saturated fat—if anything, having a lot of it over a long period of time is probably unhealthy for their heart. However, for cancer patients who are trying to build up after treatment, or just maintain their intake, it's usually fine to have a bit of coconut yoghurt, milk, cream or oil in products.

Extra virgin olive oil is a healthier fat alternative.

## Sugar and sweets

With no evidence that consuming sugar causes cancer or makes cancer cells grow faster, there is no need to restrict it altogether. However, over-consumption of sugar, particularly the added sugars in processed beverages and foods, can contribute to obesity—an important risk factor for cancer.

The best way to go is to avoid excess refined sugar, as it doesn't provide much nutritional value apart from calories.

Many foods such as bread, pasta, dairy and fruit contain carbohydrate or natural sugars that are safe to eat and break down slowly in the body. Sugar-containing foods like ice cream are fine in moderation; indeed, they can be a source of extra calories if you are losing weight.

People should always consult with their GP or a dietitian before going onto a diet high in proteins, fats and sugar, to make sure their diet is tailored to their specific needs.

For patients who have not suffered weight loss, it is still important to maintain energy levels and strength. Lean proteins, such as fish and poultry, and low-fat dairy products are ideal in these circumstances. Good ways of boosting energy levels are eating fruit with yoghurt, vegetables with dips, or snacking on nuts and dried fruits.

## Keeping food safe

When undergoing cancer treatment, it is particularly important to avoid foodborne illnesses—they sap the strength and are potentially more dangerous because of cancer's destructive effect on the immune system.

Food safety is paramount with chemo patients—things like soft cheeses and raw eggs and fish are high-risk foods for their fragile systems.

High-risk foods to avoid:

◆ raw or undercooked eggs, meat and fish

◆ soft cheeses

◆ reheated food that is not piping hot

◆ unpasteurised dairy products.

Temperature is important:

◆ Cold foods need to be straight out of the fridge.

◆ Hot foods must be cooked thoroughly, and eaten hot.

Tips for leftovers:

◆ Leftovers should be stored carefully and discarded if uneaten after a couple of days.

◆ Unused food should be refrigerated within two hours of cooking—and modern refrigerators mean that piping-hot foods don't need to cool down first.

◆ Opened cans should not be refrigerated—tin and iron will dissolve from the can walls and the food may develop a metallic taste. Tin may cause digestive problems, fever or headache.

## Changing needs

Nutritional needs transform during the cancer journey, from diagnosis through treatment, and vary with the type of treatment.

A huge number of cancer patients find that general advice is handy. However, some people need a dietitian for individualised one-on-one advice—they may be suffering things like persistent nausea and vomiting, have had bowel surgery or their tolerance of certain foods has changed, for example.

Because of these diverse needs, the recommendations in this chapter will not apply to everyone—if you're suffering a lot of symptoms that are making it hard for you to eat, talk to your health professional.

## Mixing it up

Generally, people with cancer should try to eat foods from as many different food groups—vegetables, fruit, grains, lean meats/fish and dairy—as they can face. A varied diet helps to stimulate the appetite and overcome the apathy many patients feel towards food.

What's more, eating a well-balanced diet that includes plenty of green leafy vegetables and nuts can better help you get the calcium and protein you need rather than relying too much on dairy.

While it may be tempting to augment the diet—or to believe food can be replaced to some extent—with vitamin and mineral supplements, this should be avoided. The most beneficial source of vitamins and minerals is the foods that are rich in them anyway. Another reason applies to cancer patients: high doses of vitamins can negate the effect of radiotherapy, chemotherapy and targeted therapies.

If people are already taking vitamin supplements when they are diagnosed, they should stop taking them, and at least seek advice about their supplement regime from a GP or dietitian.

## EXERCISING THE BODY

Regular exercise is important for most people with cancer. At the very least, light exercise can help to stimulate the appetite for people who are off their food or struggling with being motivated to eat. Always seek medical advice, though, before embarking on any exercise program—some cancers require a modified plan to avoid complications.

Exercise benefits everyone. A 2013 Harvard study showed that just 15 minutes of exercise a day can increase life span by as much as three years, with increasing benefits for each minute after that.

Exercise has been shown to reduce your risk of getting cancer, and many studies published by the National Cancer Institute show that cancer patients who don't exercise are more likely to die than those who exercise regularly. So one thing cancer survivors can do to lower the odds of cancer recurrence is to exercise, even at a moderate level. For example, a six-year study showed that patients with metastatic colorectal cancer who engaged in moderate exercise while undergoing chemotherapy tended to have delayed progression of their disease and fewer severe side effects from treatment. Even low-intensity exercise, such as walking four or more hours a week, was associated with almost 20% less cancer progression or death over the course of the study.

New research from Edith Cowan University shows the proteins created by the body when exercising (*myokines*) can suppress tumour growth and even help actively fight cancerous cells. Study supervisor Professor Rob Newton said the results help explain why cancer progresses more slowly in patients who exercise.

'When we took their pre-exercise blood and their post-exercise blood and placed it over living prostate cancer cells, we saw a significant suppression of the growth of those cells from the post-training blood,' he explained. 'That's quite substantial, indicating chronic [long-term, as opposed to single-session] exercise creates a cancer-suppressive environment in the body.'

Recently, Melbourne cardiologist Professor André La Gerche found that monitored exercise programs can prevent the harsh effects of toxic drugs on the cardiovascular system. He found participants showed no evidence of heart damage as a result of chemotherapy drugs.

### Kinds of exercise

Exercise gives a sense of achievement and a way of benchmarking progress during treatment, as some of the patients we met earlier in the book highlighted. Exercise also has physical benefits that help offset the side effects of treatment—it releases endorphins, which ease lethargy, fatigue and anxiety. Simply going for a walk, doing some stretches or performing basic resistance work make patients feel better in themselves, as well as improving strength and stamina. A minimum of 30 minutes a day is ideal for healthy adults, although Cancer Council Victoria advises that if you have cancer, you should be as physically active as your abilities and condition allow.

### Building stamina

Start out gradually with two or three sessions of 15 or 10 minutes each if you do not feel up to doing it all in one go. However, the amount of time you can manage in any one session quickly increases with regular exercise.

You may get sore muscles if you're starting a new form of exercise. If the soreness doesn't go away in a few days, tell your doctor.

If your cancer means you cannot lift weights or put yourself through too vigorous a program—for example, those with myeloma or other cancers that have spread to their bones—you can exercise in the pool, whether swimming or doing aqua aerobics.

## *Safety tips*

If you're going out to exercise, let someone know when you'll be back and remember to take a phone.

These symptoms are warning signs. If you notice any while you're exercising, stop immediately and, in Australia, call 000 for urgent medical help:

◆ pain or pressure in your chest

◆ pain down your arms

◆ severe shortness of breath

◆ dizziness or fainting

◆ irregular or unusually rapid heartbeat

◆ nausea and/or vomiting

◆ extreme weakness or fatigue.

## GETTING ENOUGH SLEEP

Although few of us would argue with our need to eat well and exercise, our need for good-quality sleep still isn't widely accepted, even though more than 17,000 studies have now proven numerous benefits of adequate sleep. And who wouldn't want to be happier, less depressed, less anxious, cleverer, slimmer and healthier?

Although the WHO stipulates a minimum of eight hours sleep a night for adults, whatever their age, two-thirds of adults throughout the world's developed nations don't manage to achieve this.

Neuroscientist Matthew Walker shows that if you regularly sleep less than six or seven hours a night:

◆ your immune system is 'demolished'

◆ your blood-sugar levels are 'disrupted profoundly'

◆ you're at greater risk of 'major physical and psychiatric conditions'.

Dr Michael Irwin at University of California, Los Angeles pioneered studies of the effects of even a brief dose of short sleep on cancer-fighting immune cells. In a group of healthy young men, he found that just one night of four hours of sleep swept away 70% of the immune system's circulating natural killer cells, compared to a full eight-hour sleep.

Imagine the weak state of your cancer-fighting weaponry after a week of short sleep, let alone months or even years.

## Sleep disruptors

Medications, medical conditions and any thoughts playing on your mind can affect the quality and quantity of your sleep, disrupt its timing and reduce *sleep efficiency*—the percentage of time you were asleep while in bed. Say you spend eight hours in bed and sleep right through, your sleep efficiency is 100%, but if you only sleep four hours out of eight, it works out to just 50%.

Most sleep doctors recommend 90% or above for good-quality sleep.

Sleep patterns change as we age. 'Sleep is more problematic and disordered in older adults,' says Walker. And if we believe that older people need less sleep, we're mistaken. Research finds that older adults need just as much sleep as younger people.

Research also found that low-level exhaustion caused by chronic lack of sleep actually skews people's perception of how much worse they are now functioning. As Walker says, 'You don't know how sleep-deprived you are when you are sleep-deprived.'

## 5 keys to a good sleep

If you're still having trouble sleeping after you've taken care of the following five things, talk to your GP.

1. Time: schedule your sleep time and only take naps before 3 pm.
2. Exercise: this is great, but not less than three hours before bedtime.
3. Food and drink: avoid coffee, nicotine, big meals and alcohol late at night.

4. Environment: keep your bedroom dark, cool, gadget-free, comfortable.
5. Medications: if some delay or disrupt your sleep, talk to your healthcare professional about taking them earlier in the day.

## COMPLEMENTARY MEDICINE

*Complementary therapies and medicines* focus on the whole person, rather than just the cancer. Many forms of complementary medicine can ease the symptoms of treatment and create a calm space to enable healing.

Many people living with cancer use complementary therapies—some of the most popular are mind-body therapies including art therapies, hypnosis, massage, meditation, mindfulness, relaxation and imagery, traditional Chinese medicine, and yoga.

These therapies have been found to be useful in treating common side effects—such as nausea and vomiting, pain, fatigue, anxiety and depressive symptoms—and improving overall quality of life. Some also affect biomarkers such as immune function and stress hormones.

Research is increasing into complementary therapies and medicines, and at this stage some therapies are supported by strong evidence while others lack the rigorous scientific evidence required by conventional medicines.

### *Clinically proven benefits*
These complementary therapies have been rigorously tested and shown to help in specific ways.

◆ Meditation, relaxation, counselling, support groups, massage, acupuncture, yoga, naturopathic nutrition, qi gong and t'ai chi have all been shown to improve quality of life.

◆ Meditation, relaxation, counselling, spiritual practices, massage and acupuncture can help with reducing stress, anxiety and fatigue.

◆ Acupuncture and hypnotherapy reduce chemotherapy-induced nausea and vomiting.

◆ Spiritual practices have been shown to improve the ability to manage challenges.

◆ Aromatherapy can help with relaxation and sleep.

◆ T'ai chi improves strength and flexibility.

◆ Naturopathic nutrition prevents and manages malnutrition, and helps heal wounds and damaged tissue.

◆ Massage helps with muscle tension.

◆ Art therapy and music therapy reduce anxiety and help to express feelings.

The Cancer Council recommends keeping all your healthcare providers informed to reduce the risk of any adverse reactions, especially during treatment. Some complementary therapies can affect the way conventional medicines work, and even stop them working.

### Complementary versus alternative medicine

It's important to recognise the difference between *complementary* medicine—which supports and enhances the treatment recommended by your medical team—and *alternative* practitioners who are promoting their treatment as better than conventional treatment. Complementary therapies are used *alongside* conventional treatments and medicines, usually to manage side effects. Alternative therapies are used *instead of* conventional treatments.

Many complementary therapies are being scientifically researched for use in people with cancer, while many alternative therapies have not been scientifically tested, so there is no proof they stop cancer growing or spreading. Others have been tested and shown not to be effective. While side effects of alternative treatments are not always known, some are serious and can delay or stop the cancer being treated effectively.

'Be wary of someone who says you don't need to go down that traditional path,' Alyx Stewart says.

## *Warning signs*

◆ The practitioner is not qualified through an accredited educational institution or registered with a professional organisation.

◆ The practitioner tells you that conventional medical treatment will stop their treatment from working, or asks you not to talk to your doctors about their treatment.

◆ The practitioner tells you their treatment cures cancer and says clinical studies exist to prove its effectiveness, but doesn't show you evidence in trusted medical journals.

◆ The practitioner won't tell you the ingredients in a herbal preparation they give you.

◆ The treatment costs a lot of money, you need to pay in advance for several months' treatment, or you need to travel overseas to have the treatment.

## HELPING SOMEONE WITH CANCER

When you find out a friend or a family member has cancer, it can be hard to know how to help. But try putting yourself in their place: imagine yourself suddenly in a bewildering situation where your world has been tipped upside down and your disease—not only being unwell, but also the treatment and its side effects—has hijacked your life.

'Whatever you need in your house, someone with cancer needs,' Alyx Stewart says. Think of the tasks that keep everyday life going— shopping, cooking, cleaning, home maintenance, for example.

◆ Can you drive them to appointments, or sit with them during treatment?

◆ Can you give them time, say, to read them the news or the kind of books they enjoy?

◆ Do they love music? Perhaps you can create a set-up for them to listen to it.

We decide what we eat every day, and we socialise through food. Food and nutrition give people a great sense of control.

A lot of people see they can help by bringing food and providing meals. Remember that a person with cancer has a compromised immune system. When bringing food, it's important to store or serve it safely rather than, for example, leaving it on the veranda.

## Tempting with taste and smell

Think about flavour to tempt someone to eat if they are feeling nauseous.

Research has found that 80% of what we assume to be taste is actually down to our sense of smell.

'When someone experiences smell and taste changes due to cancer treatment, we need to be sure to add additional clues to food to make it interesting for them again,' Alyx Stewart comments. 'It's not as simple as eating strong-flavoured foods.'

We have five basic tastes, she explains: sweet, sour, salty, bitter and umami. *Umami* is that savouriness that we can't quite put our finger on, but makes food taste even better.

Smell is integral to flavour perception and by layering smells with the use of carefully chosen ingredients, we can stimulate the appetite.

We also need to consider how food feels in the mouth using different textures. In the absence of taste, we need other clues to add interest in eating again.

The *trigeminal nerve* is important for detecting the 'heat' in chilli and wasabi, and the coolness of foods like mint. Adding ingredients that stimulate the trigeminal nerve gives clues that there is something going on in the mouth, even if we cannot taste it fully. Again, it is about making food interesting enough to eat.

Combine umami, texture, smell and trigeminal nerve stimulation, and make a dish with several 'layers' of interest to stimulate the appetite and add excitement to mealtimes.

### Helpful tips

There are no set rules and every friendship is different—think about your unique relationship and let that guide you. Often the little things mean the most.

Remember to ask permission before visiting, offering advice or asking questions.

Still stuck for ways to support your friend or family member? An internet search will throw up useful apps and suggestions.

## PALLIATIVE CARE

Our patient stories underline how debilitating cancer can be, but also how being as strong as possible helps the body to fight the disease. In all the different forms of treatment palliative measures—those that manage pain and relieve the symptoms of the disease—are crucial in helping patients combat their cancer.

More and more treatment centres now offer comprehensive palliative care—also known as supportive care—teams that help patients in a number of ways. They offer advice on nutrition and exercise, and provide counselling to help patients and their families deal with the mental anguish of a cancer diagnosis and cope with surgery, radiotherapy, chemotherapy or whatever treatments are prescribed to fight the disease. The teams also offer practical information on how to manage the financial aspects of treatment and day-to-day living expenses when a patient's work life is interrupted.

Along with good nutrition, appropriate exercise and a positive mental approach, palliative care can improve quality of life and increase life expectancy.

For those with curable forms of cancer, improving general health and reducing stress improves the chances of curative treatment being successful.

For those whose forms of cancer are currently incurable, being stronger and not giving up can extend life expectancy—this increases the likelihood of a cure being found in the near future while they can still benefit from it.

# SURVIVORSHIP

As we have seen throughout this book, breakthroughs in cancer screening, detection and treatment have been monumental. And that means a rapid increase in the number of people surviving cancer.

Survival rates after a cancer diagnosis are on the increase with the latest figures showing nearly 70% of people are alive after five years, up from less than 50% in the 1980s. In 2020, it was estimated that there were just under 150,000 new cases of cancer diagnosed and just under 50,000 deaths from cancer.

This adds up to a lot of survivors. A cancer survivor, defined broadly, is a person at any stage between diagnosis and the remainder of their life, so they may be a cancer patient awaiting or undergoing treatment or between treatments, or moving, post-treatment, from being a cancer patient to a cancer survivor.

It isn't necessarily smooth sailing being pronounced free of cancer. People may still experience problems—side effects, pain, fatigue, disrupted sleep, changed body functions, foggy thinking, fears of cancer returning—as well as changed relationships and financial status.

The best way to manage this is by taking control of your own health and learning how to cope with the changes or issues that you may experience during and after your cancer treatment.

Changing lifestyle behaviours can help to improve quality of life, manage side effects, reduce the risk of your cancer coming back, and prevent new health issues from occurring:

◆ improving eating habits

◆ reducing alcohol consumption

◆ increasing exercise

◆ quitting smoking

◆ reducing sun exposure.

Taking control of your own health means monitoring it:

◆ recognising symptoms that may require looking into before your next scheduled appointment

◆ keeping your appointments

◆ having regular, scheduled check-ups.

Best of all, with this growing cohort of survivors comes support—your GP, cancer treatment team, Cancer Australia or, internationally, World Health Organization, and a network of community and non-government organisations right around the world.

## MANAGING PAIN

Professor Melanie Lovell is a leading palliative medicine physician and founding Chair of the Australian Cancer Pain Management Guideline Working Party. She says about half of all people who survive cancer face ongoing pain.

'Living with cancer presents lots of challenges,' she says. 'Experiencing pain as well places an additional burden on top of what may be a difficult experience.'

Professor Lovell says the best pain control involves clinicians and the person living with cancer collaborating on approaches that combine medicines with evidence-based approaches that don't involve drugs.

While opioid drugs are effective for relief at end-of-life, those who are living with chronic pain need other evidence-based approaches to manage their pain.

Some techniques use the mind to manage pain, such as applying gate control theory, harnessing the power of neuroplasticity, retraining the nervous system, meditation and mindfulness. Those that use the body include exercise, such as strength training and stretching for managing pain, and learning how to relax.

◆ ◆ ◆

Although, as we have seen in this book, our genetic make-up—and mutations in it—are a key factor in whether or not we develop cancer, it is becoming increasingly clear that how we live our lives can also influence whether or not we develop the disease.

## CANCER RISKS

While it is still too early to link specific foods to increased cancer risk, there is growing evidence that too much salt can damage the lining of the stomach, which makes it vulnerable to cancer-causing carcinogens, and a diet over-reliant on red and processed meats leads to a higher risk of developing pancreatic cancer.

Alcohol use causes 3% of cancers, says Cancer Council Australia. The level of risk of developing an alcohol-related cancer increases in line with the level of consumption. Evidence shows that alcohol use increases the risk of cancers of the mouth, pharynx, larynx, oesophagus, stomach, bowel, liver and breast.

Even worse, alcohol use may contribute to greater body fatness, linked to cancers of the oesophagus, pancreas, gallbladder, stomach, bowel, endometrium, ovary, kidney, liver, breast in post-menopausal women, and prostate.

Lung cancer is responsible for the most cancer deaths every year, and the link between it and smoking is irrefutable.

Together, smoking and alcohol have a synergistic effect on cancer risk, multiplying into a far greater risk than the sum of the two.

Healthy lifestyle choices are, therefore, important in the fight against cancer for those both with and without the disease. The vast amount of investment, time and expertise that has gone into producing the breakthroughs we have learned about in this book will continue. It is up to all of us to support those who are doing that work.

# Chapter 12

# HOW TO EAT WELL

Sometimes we love to cook. That's when it's fun to spend hours sourcing, preparing, cooking and plating up. And sometimes we don't. Cancer can have a lot to do with that, whether it's the treatment or the symptoms. Too often we stop enjoying food and find it hard to eat.

Yet the body must have fuel to repair itself.

In this chapter we will explore:

◆ how to load up every morsel with nutrition

◆ basics to stock up on

◆ some simple ideas for good eating.

No research has shown that any particular eating plan can prevent or cure cancer. And there are no particular foods you should eat if you have cancer.

The crucial thing is to pack nutrition into every bite, especially if your appetite is low.

The best way to manage is to eat small and often, whether hungry or not. And whether the hardest thing is deciding what to cook or getting supplies in, planning ahead is the way to go.

If you are undergoing chemotherapy, you will have changing symptoms and ability to eat, depending on where you are between the chemo cycles. Planning meals across the cycles will help. You may not feel like cooking during the weeks of your treatment, so consider making some meals ahead and freezing them. If family and friends can arrange a meal roster, this will really help.

What you put into your body will enhance your quality of life whether you're fit and well, a person with or recovering from cancer, or a cancer survivor.

Here are some ideas for stocking up.

## GOOD EATING—THE BASICS

Check our basics lists for some ideas on staples to have on hand so there's always something simple, succulent and, above all, nutritious in the pantry or freezer. For example, when you look in the fridge and find some cheese, you'll know you can build it into a meal. And melted cheese works wonders to add to taste.

### *10 things for the pantry*

1.  Fish: cans of salmon, sardines, tuna
2.  Pulses: cans of beans, lentils, chickpeas
3.  Vegetables: cans of tomatoes, mushrooms
4.  Fruit: cans or jars with no added sugar
5.  Oats: steel cut and traditional rolled are better than instant
6.  Pasta: an assortment of shapes
7.  Quinoa: whole or flakes
8.  Rice: arborio, basmati, brown, wild rice
9.  Herbs and spices: start with Italian herbs, parsley, chilli, anise, cinnamon
10. Nuts and seeds: almonds, pistachios, walnuts, Brazil nuts; flaxseeds, chia, hemp and sunflower seeds

### *7 things for the freezer*

Your freezer is your best friend. Make sure to mark frozen items with the date to use by—masking tape and a waterproof pen will do the trick.

**Tip:** Make a simple marinade and coat chicken fillets or pieces before freezing. The chicken will marinate as it defrosts.

1.  Protein: beef, chicken, fish, lamb, pork, tofu
2.  Vegetables: riced cauliflower, peas, spinach, sweet corn, medleys
3.  Bread: wholegrain or wholemeal slices or rolls
4.  Fruit: berries and cherries
5.  Cheeses: cooking cheeses like Cheddar and mozzarella freeze best

6. Ice cream
7. Juices (as icy poles)

## *Tips to help side effects*

◆ Bread is really good if you need something soft and palatable.

◆ Herbs and spices add flavour to bland foods—the quantity can be adjusted depending on how you are feeling.

◆ Balsamic vinegar zaps up sliced avocado or tomato.

◆ Protein—chicken, fish, meat, quinoa, pulses like chickpeas, lentils, beans, split peas—will stave off muscle wastage.

◆ Cruciferous vegetables—cauliflower, cabbage, garden cress, bok choy, broccoli, Brussels sprouts—are powerhouses of nutrition. Try mixing riced cauliflower 50:50 with rice to up your nutrients and fibre.

◆ Nuts make the perfect snack, as long as you can swallow. Keep them in the fridge for maximum goodness.

◆ Salads make a great one-bowl meal combining protein, grains, vegetables and nuts. Our dietician suggests grains with a combination of protein, whether it's quinoa, or brown rice with beans, plus chickpeas and lentils, if people can manage them. 'And cheese,' she adds—perhaps grated tasty cheese or different kinds such as feta or ricotta.

◆ Find the freshest fruit and veg in markets—organic can be better, but use your common sense and go by look, feel and taste. Even better, grow your own!

◆ For nausea, apple, ginger, banana, lemon and peppermint work well—stock up on fresh fruit, jars of mixed ginger, peppermint tea, and lemon spices like lemon pepper.

◆ For a sore mouth, lasagne is great, whether based on meat or pulses. It can be easily frozen as single meals, too. Make sure to include lots of cancer-fighting vegetables such as tomatoes, garlic and carrot. And custard soothes tender membranes too.

# SIMPLE RECIPES FOR GOOD EATING

Once you're stocked up, it's easy to start off with what you have at hand and build it into a meal or snack.

Here's a breakdown of the recipe ideas and where you'll find them.

## 6 ways with smoothies

Smoothies are a brilliant way to pack nutrition into a form that's easy to get down for people suffering from low appetite or side effects that make the mouth sensitive.

The combinations are endless—you can make up whatever you like from the basic components. Vary your ingredients according to season, mood and any side effects—add other proteins, fruits, vegetables, nuts and seeds and extra fibre.

### Tips

◆ Chia seeds are a good gluten-free choice for fibre, protein, calcium, omega-3 fatty acids and other minerals. Ideal for vegans.

◆ Other milks such as hemp, almond, coconut, cashew and rice don't measure up to dairy and soy milks in terms of protein, although calcium is often added.

◆ It's worth checking alternative milks for the addition of cane sugar. They may be valuable for other nutrients such as Vitamin D, omega and amino acids.

◆ Also check protein powders for added sugar and multiple ingredients.

◆ Fresh fruit is usually better than juices, which may contain as much sugar as commercial soft drinks.

◆ Dates sweeten without empty calories—they're packed with antioxidants, fibre and potassium.

### 1. Smoothie 101

*1 serve*

Protein (2 tablespoons): almond meal, vegan protein powder, oats, quinoa powder, chia seeds, eggs or nuts
Fibre (1 tablespoon): psyllium husk, flax or wheatgerm
Fruits or vegetables (1–2 pieces or 1 cup: frozen and/or fresh)

Liquid (1 cup): dairy or soy, or a mixture of milk and yoghurt
Healthy fats (1 teaspoon): coconut oil or ½ avocado, to taste

**METHOD**

For one-step smoothies, a heavy-duty blender will chop up things like frozen fruit. Or you can mash up bananas, defrost frozen berries overnight, and add it all to a shaker.

### 2. Banana and berry

Add **1 large banana** and **½ cup berries** to your choice of protein, fibre, liquid and healthy fats.

### 3. Peach, strawberry and almond

Add **1 peach, ½ cup strawberries, ¼ cup sliced or slivered almonds** and **¼ teaspoon ground ginger or cinnamon** to your choice of liquid.

### 4. Avocado, feta and orange

Add **½ ripe avocado, 50g feta cheese, 1 orange** and **¼ teaspoon ground cinnamon or cardamom** to your choice of liquid.

**Tip:** Make sure feta smells sweet and has been open no more than three days.

### 5. Apple and berry

Add **1 apple, ½ cup berries, juice of ½ lemon** and **1 tablespoon honey** to your choice of protein, fibre, liquid and healthy fats.

### 6. Chia and berry

Add **2 tablespoons chia seeds, ½ cup blueberries or strawberries** and **1–2 drops pure vanilla** to your choice of liquid. More protein, fibre, healthy fats and sweetener are optional.

This goes particularly well with yoghurt. You don't have to soak chia seeds, but if you have 15 minutes to soak them in your chosen liquid until they swell up, it will give a lovely soft texture.

## 10 ways with porridge

Porridge is packed with fibre, antioxidants, vitamins, minerals and healthy fats, as well as protein, which you can boost by cooking the oats with quinoa or chia and adding nuts to serve.

The oat kernels burst open during cooking, giving creaminess and sweetness that goes beautifully with fruit, seeds, nuts, yoghurt and maple syrup or honey. Cream adds extra energy to fortify food when you're trying to build up weight and strength. Stevia is an alternative sweetener with almost no calories.

Least to most processed are steel cut, rolled or quick oats, with cooking times of 40, 15 and several minutes, respectively. Quick oats have more additives for flavour and creaminess.

**Tip**: Cook several servings of steel cut or rolled oats and refrigerate in serving-size containers to reheat, adding water as needed.

### 1. Porridge 101

*2 serves*

50g rolled oats
Pinch of sea salt
400ml milk, soy milk and/or water

**METHOD**

Place the oats in a saucepan with milk and/or water.

Heat to boiling over medium heat then turn down heat to very low and simmer for 4–5 minutes, stirring so it doesn't stick to the bottom. It's cooked when it's creamy. (If it does stick, turn off the heat, put on the lid and leave it for a couple of minutes, then stir.)

Serving ideas:

◆ Yoghurt for fermented nutrition

◆ Honey or maple syrup for sweetening

◆ Milk, soy milk or yoghurt whey for liquid

◆ Psyllium husk, bran flakes, chia seeds or flaxseeds for fibre

◆ Stewed, fresh or frozen fruit for vitamins, minerals, antioxidants and fibre

**Tip:** Shorten cooking time by covering the oats with cold water the night before. Or add boiling water and cook immediately.

### 2. Winter warmer

Cook **porridge 101** and when almost done, stir in **2 tablespoons dried fruit** (raisins, currants, sultanas, apricots etc) and **1 teaspoon coconut oil**.

### 3. Greek island

Cook **porridge 101** and serve, topped with **1–2 teaspoons honey, 2–4 tablespoons yoghurt** and **1 tablespoon chopped almonds**.

### 4. Chia and pear

Soak **20g chia seeds** in **1 cup water** for 20 minutes. Cook **porridge 101**. As it cooks, slice **1 pear** into a small saucepan. Add **2 tablespoons maple syrup** and cook it over low heat until soft, or leave it raw. Add chia seeds to porridge, stirring, and heat for just long enough to see bubbles begin to form. Serve porridge with pear slices arranged on top and maple syrup or cooking juices drizzled over.

### 5. Banana, blueberry and pecan

Cook **porridge 101**. Slice **1 large banana** into it and allow it to heat through. Toast **1 tablespoon pecans** and break them into pieces. Serve porridge with **½ cup fresh or thawed blueberries** and sprinkle over pecans.

### 6. Crunchy granola and apple

Cook **porridge 101**. Serve sprinkled with **¼ cup granola (toasted muesli), 1 sliced or grated** apple and **milk or cream** to taste.

**Tip:** Use quinoa flakes and add boiling water to oats and quinoa flakes. Leave 5 minutes, then bring to the boil and cook for 2–3 minutes.

### 7. Banana, coconut, vanilla and kiwifruit

Cook **porridge 101**. Stir in **¼ teaspoon pure vanilla extract** and **2 tablespoons shredded coconut**. Smash **1 large banana** through and serve with **2 sliced kiwifruit** and extra **coconut**.

### 8. Quinoa, banana, sultanas and cinnamon

Place **20g quinoa, 30g oats, ½ teaspoon cinnamon** and **400ml water, milk or soy milk** in a saucepan. Bring to the boil, stir as it thickens, then leave to simmer for an extra 10 minutes with the lid on. Add **1 tablespoon sultanas** and **1 large sliced banana** and allow them to heat through. Serve with a swirl of **1 tablespoon honey**.

### 9. Honeyed apple, walnuts and vanilla

Cook **porridge 101**. Meanwhile, toast and roughly chop **1 tablespoon walnuts**. Core and slice **2 red apples** and cook with **2 tablespoons honey** over low heat until translucent. Stir **¼ teaspoon pure vanilla extract** into porridge and serve topped with apple and walnuts and drizzled with cooking juice.

### 10. Porridge pikelets

Preheat the oven to 100°C. Beat **1 egg** in a large bowl then add **200g/1 cup leftover porridge** and mix well. Add **½ teaspoon ground cinnamon** and **50g/½ cup dried fruit**. Heat **1 tablespoon coconut oil, butter or ghee** in a medium frying pan until hot but not smoking. Space 4 tablespoonsful of batter around the pan and cook till golden, about 4 minutes. Flip over carefully and in about 3 minutes, when golden, remove, stack on a plate and keep warm in the oven. Add **1 tablespoon coconut oil, butter or ghee** and cook the last four pikelets. Serve stacked with **fruit, yoghurt** and **honey or maple syrup**.

## *1001 ways with a can of soup*

You'll find some delicious choices in the canned soup aisle—just the ticket if you need something quick, warming and easy on the throat.

The trick here is to start with the healthiest soup possible. Check the nutrition information:

◆ Is it low in sodium? Less than 450mg per serving is ideal.

◆ How much sugar does it contain?

◆ Is the ingredients list short, containing natural foods?

Go for natural ingredients you know rather than a lot of chemical names you don't recognise.

Now build it up into nourishing, flavourful goodness by adding proteins, healthy fats, vegetables, herbs and spices, and sides.

Protein:

◆ diced chicken

◆ seared tofu

◆ chopped hard-boiled eggs

◆ beaten eggs

◆ beans

◆ yoghurt

Vegetables:

◆ crisped-up kale or sautéed green veg

◆ leftover roast vegetables

◆ fresh or frozen vegetables simmered until cooked

Multigrain or wholemeal bread or toast:

◆ on the side

◆ made into garlic croutons

Cheese:

◆ grated tasty or Parmesan cheese

◆ crumbled feta or goat cheese

◆ shredded mozzarella

Fats:

◆ swirl of extra-virgin olive oil

◆ an avocado

◆ sour cream

Nuts, toasted:

◆ almond slivers

◆ pine nuts

◆ walnuts

Seeds:

◆ pumpkin

◆ sunflower

◆ chia

◆ sesame

## 10 ways with cheese

Cheese is handy as a snack, whether it's cheese on toast or cream cheese with crackers, cheese and biscuits, melted cheese and scrambled eggs. It can be used as a staple, but is also a good fortifier.

Beware of high-risk soft cheeses such as brie, camembert, ricotta and feta—make sure they haven't been opened for more than three days.

### 1. Welsh rarebit

*2 serves*

40g butter or olive-oil spread
50g plain flour
¼ cup apple cider (or stout or milk)
1 egg, beaten
200g cheddar, grated
½ teaspoon hot English mustard
1 teaspoon sweet paprika
4 slices bread

**METHOD**

Preheat grill to high. Melt butter in a small saucepan over low heat. Whisk in flour and then stir for one minute. Add cider, stout or milk and turn heat up to medium, stirring constantly until it thickens to a paste. Remove from heat and add egg, cheddar, mustard and paprika, then return to heat and stir until it's thick and smooth—about 2 minutes. Meanwhile, toast the bread. Spoon the cheese sauce evenly over the toast, right to the edges. Place under the grill and cook till it is browned.

### 2. Buck rarebit

Top the rarebit with a **poached or fried egg**.

### 3. Blushing bunny

Add **tomato passata or soup** to the cheese sauce.

### 4. Paul's cheese on toast

For 1 serve, heat the grill. On a board, butter **2 slices wholemeal or multigrain toast** with **butter or olive-oil spread**. Arrange on it **2 thin slices onion, ¼ sliced capsicum** and **1 sliced tomato**. Season with **salt and pepper**. Cover with **slices of tasty cheese** and sprinkle over **¼ teaspoon hot English mustard powder**. Grill until melty and brown. *Also yummy made in a sandwich press.*

### 5. Spanish cheese/ tomato tosta

Preheat the grill. Lightly toast **2 slices rustic bread**. Cut **1 garlic clove** in half and rub it over the bread, then slice **2 ripe tomatoes** and add. Drizzle with **olive oil** and arrange **6 slices Manchego cheese** on top. Grill until melty and brown.

### 6. Roasted veg and cheese sauce

For 2 serves, roast **enough vegetables for 2** and keep warm. Melt **2 tablespoons butter or olive-oil spread** in a saucepan over medium heat then whisk in **2 tablespoons flour** and cook for 1 minute. Slowly pour in **350ml milk**, stirring constantly. When it is thick, add **pepper, chilli and/or other herbs or spices** to taste. Remove from the heat and gradually stir in, by handfuls, **1 cup grated sharp cheddar cheese**, waiting till each amount melts before adding more. Pour the sauce over the vegetables and serve immediately.

*This is nice on a sore mouth and can also be made with vegan cheeses.*

### 7. Baked potato with cheese sauce

For 2 serves, pour **1 quantity cheese sauce** (see recipe 6) over **2 large baked potatoes**. Drizzle over the top **salsa, chutney or sauce** to taste.

### 8. Margherita 'pizza' on flatbread

For 1 serve, preheat the oven to 180°C. Crush **1 garlic clove** and mix with **2 tablespoons olive oil**. Brush mixture over **1 piece pita or naan**, reserving what's left. Place in the oven for 5–7 minutes until crispy. Remove from the oven and top with **3 slices mozzarella cheese** then **1 sliced tomato**. Season with **salt and pepper** and **dried Italian**

**herbs** (optional). Return to the oven for 10 minutes, until edges are golden and cheese is melted. Meanwhile, add remaining oil and garlic to **balsamic vinegar** to taste. Remove the 'pizza' from the oven and drizzle with oil/balsamic mixture, and a handful of **chopped fresh basil** (optional).

*Alyx Stewart suggests this is great in the third week of treatment, especially for a sore mouth.*

### 9. Cheddar and avocado
For 2 serves, slice **1 avocado** and arrange it over **4 slices multigrain bread**. Season to taste with **black pepper** and a **squeeze of lemon juice**. Lay **6 slices vintage cheddar** over the top and serve.

### 10. Marinated feta on toast
For 2 serves, spread **½ ripe avocado** on **4 slices multigrain toast** and top with **3 tablespoons marinated feta**. Plate up with **1 bunch cooked asparagus, 12 cherry tomatoes** and **2 handfuls baby spinach** on the side. Drizzle asparagus with **1 tablespoon good olive oil** and grind **black pepper** over. Sprinkle the tomatoes and spinach with **1 tablespoon balsamic vinegar**.

## 6 ways with a can of fish

### 1. Tuna and pea pasta

For 2 serves, boil enough water for pasta in a large saucepan.
Meanwhile, heat the oil from a **185g can of tuna in oil** in a small
saucepan over medium heat. Add **1 small to medium chopped onion**,
and fry until transparent. Put **170g short pasta** (fusilli works well) on
to cook. Add the tuna to the onion pan, stirring to break it up, then add
**¼ teaspoon red chilli flakes** and **black pepper** to taste. When pasta is
almost cooked, stir **1 cup frozen peas** into the tuna mixture and heat
through, then add **a splash of pasta-cooking water** and **a squeeze of
lemon** to the tuna mixture. Drain pasta and serve in bowls topped with
tuna sauce and **grated parmesan**. A small salad of **baby spinach, red
capsicum and tomatoes** is a delicious side.

### 2. Tuna mornay

For 2 serves, hard-boil **2 eggs** then cool in cold water, peel and slice.
Preheat the oven to 180°C. Grease a 1L ovenproof dish. Slice **1 small
onion** finely. Melt **20g butter or olive-oil spread** in a medium casserole
pot over low heat. Add the onion and cook till translucent. Add
**1 tablespoon plain flour** and mix, stirring, then add a little of **1½–2
cups milk**, stirring until it thickens. Gradually add the rest of the milk,
stirring, and then **185g can tuna in springwater**, drained, the **juice of
½ small lemon, 1 tablespoon breadcrumbs**, hardboiled eggs, **black
pepper** and **1 tablespoon grated tasty cheese**. Sprinkle **1 tablespoon
grated tasty cheese** on top and bake for 15 minutes, or until cheese
is melted and golden. Optional extras: cooked macaroni, diced carrot,
frozen sweetcorn or peas, crumb or mashed-potato topping, a pinch of
chilli.

### 3. Sardine sandwich

For 2 serves, chop finely **¼ small red onion or 1 spring onion** and load
onto **2 slices of bread or toast** with **110g can drained sardines, black
pepper** and a **handful of baby spinach**. Top with another **2 slices of
bread or toast**. Optional: butter the bread if the sardines aren't in oil.

### 4. Salmon fish cakes

For 2 serves, drain a **210g can salmon** and remove skin and large bones. Flake into **250g mashed potatoes**. Add **1 tablespoon chopped parsley** and season with **salt and pepper**. Mix well and form into four cakes. Place in a shallow bowl **2 tablespoons plain flour** and coat cakes, shaking off excess as you go. Heat **2 tablespoons olive oil** in a frypan and cook cakes over medium heat for 3–4 minutes each side until golden and heated through. Serve with **lemon wedges**. Optional extras: add finely chopped onion to the mix; coat cakes with 1 beaten egg and ¼ cup breadcrumbs after the flour—you may need extra oil for this.

### 5. White bean and tuna salad

For 4 serves, shake in a jar with lid **50ml olive oil**, **35ml red wine vinegar**, **1 crushed garlic clove** and **1 teaspoon Dijon mustard**. Drain and rinse a **400g can cannellini beans**, place them in a bowl and fork in the tuna from a **225g can tuna in oil**, with a little oil from the can. Finely chop **1 small red onion** and add it with **1 handful black olives**, and **2–3 chopped anchovy fillets**. Chop and add **1 handful basil or oregano** and **1 handful flatleaf parsley**. Pour over the dressing and mix.

### 6. Sardines, potatoes and pine nuts

For 2 serves, lightly toast **30g pine nuts** in a heavy-based frying pan and reserve for later. Scrub **400g potatoes** and cut into bite-size pieces. Heat **1 tablespoon olive oil** and add the potatoes, browning them over moderate heat for a good 15 minutes, stirring every so often. Meanwhile, finely dice 1 **small onion or 3 spring onions**, then add to the frying pan and cook till translucent. Roughly chop **3 tablespoons parsley** and stir it in with the pine nuts and 1 can sardines in olive oil.

## 10 ways with meatballs

Meatballs are a great way to get some protein in. 'They're snack size, so for people who don't have a huge appetite they're quite a good option,' our nutritionist advised. Make up a batch and cook them all—they freeze well.

### 1. Meatballs 101

30g butter or olive-oil spread
1 onion, finely chopped
1 teaspoon herbes de provence or dried marjoram, oregano and basil
Salt and black pepper
400g beef
1 egg
1–2 garlic cloves, minced (optional)
3 tablespoons olive oil
Parsley to serve

**METHOD**

Melt the butter or olive-oil spread in a frying pan over low heat, add the onion and cook for 5 minutes or until transparent. Stir in the herb blend and salt. In a bowl, add the onions to the mince, egg and garlic if using. Mix with your hands. Shape into 12 balls. Heat the olive oil in the frying pan over medium heat. Add the meatballs and cook, turning often, for 15 minutes until golden brown. Serve garnished with parsley, with salad or vegetables.

### 2. Baked

Preheat the oven to 220°C fan-forced. Grease a baking dish with butter or oil, then place the meatballs in it. Reduce heat to 120°C and bake for 30 minutes or until cooked through.

### 3. Indian

Replace the butter with **ghee** and replace the herbs with **a curry leaf and ground cumin, turmeric and fenugreek** to taste.

### 4. Mexican

Replace the herbs with **ground cumin, sweet paprika and a dash of cayenne pepper**.

### 5. Greek

Replace the herbs with **finely chopped oregano** and serve with **lemon wedges**.

### 6. Bocconcini

Press a **baby bocconcini** into the centre of each meatball.

### 7. Lamb and feta

Replace beef with **lamb** and press a cube of **feta** into the centre of each meatball.

### 8. Chicken and lettuce wraps

Replace beef mince with **chicken mince**. Wrap cooked meatballs in **lettuce** and serve with **dips or dressing** (sweet chilli sauce, chutney, pickles etc).

### 9. Pork meatballs

Replace beef mince with **pork mince** and double the herb quantity—choose sweet paprika, dried thyme, coriander and/or cumin.

### 10. Spaghetti

Make 24 meatballs instead of 12. Cook as usual then heat through in a **tomato-based pasta sauce** as spaghetti is cooking.

## 6 ways for vegetarians

### 1. Hummus

400g can of chickpeas, drained and rinsed

2 garlic cloves, crushed

2 teaspoons ground cumin

Pinch of cayenne

2–3 tablespoons lemon juice

2 tablespoons tahini (optional)

¼ teaspoon paprika

Sprigs of parsley

2–3 tablespoons olive oil

METHOD

In a blender, process chickpeas, garlic, cumin, cayenne, lemon juice and tahini if using, tasting as you go for a balanced yet sharp taste. Add a little water and blend to a creamy purée. Spoon onto a plate and drizzle with oil, then sprinkle over paprika, garnish with parsley and serve with wholemeal pita and vegetable sticks.

### 2. White bean dip

400g can cannellini beans, drained and rinsed

2 garlic cloves, chopped

2 teaspoons rosemary, chopped

½ lemon, juiced

25ml olive oil

Salt and black pepper

6–12 Kalamata olives

Handful baby spinach

½ red pepper, cut into strips

Crusty or flatbread

METHOD

Purée the beans, garlic, rosemary, lemon juice and oil until creamy and smooth. Season to taste. Serve for grazing with olives, baby spinach, red pepper and bread.

### 3. Pumpkin and sweetcorn soup

*6–10 serves*

1.5kg pumpkin, chopped into chunks
500g frozen sweetcorn
1 onion, diced
3 garlic cloves, crushed
1L chicken stock
Black pepper, ground
Chilli powder
1 tablespoon ricotta cheese per serving

**METHOD**

Place pumpkin, sweetcorn, onion, garlic and stock into a slow cooker and cook on low for 7 hours. Blend and add pepper and chilli powder to taste. Spoon ricotta over soup to serve. If cooking on stovetop, heat a little olive oil gently in a large saucepan and cook onion and garlic till transparent. Add pumpkin, sweetcorn and stock, then bring to the boil, turn heat down and cook for 40 minutes. Blend and season. To make a meal: add some protein halfway through cooking time with a can of drained and rinsed cannellini beans or chickpeas.

### 4. Salads

One-bowl salads that combine protein, grains and vegetables are easy and quick—remember to include an egg, cheese and/or a can of white, kidney or black beans, quinoa, chickpeas or lentils. Our dietician says: 'Some people find lentils or beans gassy, but if they can tolerate them okay then they're a good alternative for a vegan or vegetarian as well.'

### 5. Lentil salad

*6–8 serves*

375g brown or Puy lentils, washed
½ cup olive oil
1 onion, chopped
3 garlic cloves, chopped
½ cup fresh parsley
1 tablespoon red wine vinegar
1 tablespoon extra-virgin olive oil
Salt and black pepper

**METHOD**

Soak lentils for 2 hours. Drain, reserving 1 cup soaking water.
Heat olive oil in a medium saucepan and cook onion and garlic
until translucent. Add lentils and reserved soaking water. Cook for
20 minutes, stirring often, until lentils are cooked and water has
evaporated. Place in a bowl and add remaining ingredients. Dress it up
with hard-boil eggs or finely slice red onion or sauté extra vegetables
separately and add to the lentils in the bowl. This freezes well in single
serves (freeze without adding parsley).

## Many ways for a sweet hit

Easy, nutritious and delicious—what's not to like? These are simple to make and an alternative to readymade sweets, but without the additives.

### 1. Custard

1 tablespoon cornflour
1 tablespoon sugar or equivalent sweetener
500ml milk or half milk and cream
2 eggs
1–2 drops pure vanilla essence

**METHOD**

In a heatproof bowl, whisk cornflour and sugar with ¼ cup of milk to make a paste. Break in eggs and beat to combine. Heat remainder of milk with vanilla in a medium saucepan until hot but not boiling.

Whisk the milk into the cornflour mixture, then return to the saucepan and stir over low heat until it thickens enough to coat the back of a spoon.

### 4 Ideas to fortify custard

◆ add cinnamon or nutmeg and sliced banana

◆ soak Italian finger biscuits to soften

◆ use ground rice instead of cornflour—good with stewed prunes

◆ add ice cream or yoghurt and stewed fruit

### 2. Bread and butter pudding

*4–6 serves*

6 slices stale bread
4 teaspoons butter or olive-oil spread
60g dried fruit
2 eggs

1 tablespoon sugar or equivalent sweetener

½ teaspoon nutmeg, cinnamon or vanilla

500ml milk

2 tablespoons coconut or brown sugar (optional)

METHOD

Butter bread on one side and cut into triangles. Arrange half overlapping in a greased 1.1L oven dish, buttered side down, then sprinkle over half the dried fruit. Cover with the rest of the bread, buttered side up, and sprinkle with the rest of the fruit. Beat together eggs, sweetener, spice and milk. Pour over bread, pushing bread down to soak it up. Leave in the fridge anywhere from 2 hours to overnight. Sprinkle over coconut or brown sugar if using then bake at 180°C for 30–40 minutes until it is browned and set. *Great for breakfast as well!*

### 3. Cherry clafoutis

*4 serves*

3 eggs, beaten

¼ teaspoon vanilla

40g sugar or equivalent sweetener

40g wholemeal flour

200ml milk

400g cherries, defrosted and drained or fresh, pitted

3 tablespoons shredded coconut

Icing sugar to dust

METHOD

Preheat the oven to 190°C/180°C fan-forced, then place a 1.1L baking dish inside. Beat together eggs, vanilla, sweetener and flour, then gradually add milk, whisking to keep smooth. Remove the dish from the oven and grease or spray with olive-oil spray. Add the cherries, sprinkle over the coconut, pour over the batter then bake for 30 minutes until it is golden and set. Dust with icing sugar and serve. *This delicious French pudding is oh-so-easy.*

**Tip:**

◆ cream makes a lush addition: use 150ml milk and 50ml cream

◆ grapes and aniseed: substitute grapes for cherries and substitute 1 teaspoon fennel seeds for coconut

◆ cherries and chocolate: smash up 3–6 squares of dark chocolate and substitute for coconut

### 4. Stewed fruit 101

500g fruit (try apples, plums, pears, apricots or berries)
2 teaspoons sugar or other sweetener
2 tablespoons water

**METHOD**

Chop up all the fruit, discarding any stones, place it in a lidded saucepan with sweetener and water. Cook over medium heat until fruit has softened, then remove lid so the liquid reduces. Consistency should be quite thick.

**Tip:** Stewed fruit adds flavour and texture to porridge, yoghurt, pancakes, cereal, muesli, custard—even to a roast! Seasonal combos that work well:

◆ apple/pear

◆ rhubarb/ginger (add 50% more sweetener and grate peeled ginger into pan)

◆ feijoa/apple/ginger

### 5. Crumbles

150g plain wholemeal flour
90g brown sugar
1 teaspoon ground ginger
90g rolled oats
225g butter or olive-oil spread, melted
2 cups stewed fruit

**METHOD**

Heat the oven to 190°C. Mix the flour, sugar, ginger, oats and butter in a bowl to form crumbs. Place the stewed fruit in a small ovenproof dish and cover it with the crumble mixture. Bake for around 20 minutes (longer if the fruit has been in the fridge) until the top is golden and cooked through.

### 6. Mash-ups on bread or toast

◆ banana with honey

◆ peanut butter with raisins

◆ cream cheese with dried apricots, cranberries and sultanas

## 6 ideas for a low-fibre diet

If your doctor prescribes a low-fibre diet, perhaps before a colonoscopy or certain surgery, they will be aiming to give your digestive system a rest by restricting the amount of fibre you eat.

Only follow this diet under doctor's instructions—a low-fibre diet is made up of foods like white bread, ice cream and protein, which you shouldn't eat in large quantities, or depend on health-wise. They don't have the essential nutrients that fruits, vegetables, nuts, pulses and wholegrains contain. You'll be fine as long as the low-fibre diet is only for a short amount of time.

A doctor may stipulate no vegetables except potato and pumpkin, and only white rice, pasta and bread, with proteins such as meat, chicken, fish, eggs and cheese, as well as yoghurt, small amounts of butter and oil, and dairy if tolerated. Raw bananas and peeled, well-cooked fruit and vegetables may be allowed. Individual instructions vary, though. It's best to check your doctor's instructions.

Here are some ideas for tasty eating.

### Breakfast scrambled eggs
2 eggs
50ml milk or water
Salt to taste
Pinch of mustard powder
1 teaspoon butter or olive-oil spread
Buttered white toast

METHOD

Beat eggs, milk or water, salt and mustard powder in a bowl until blended. Heat butter in a small saucepan over medium heat until foaming. Pour in egg mixture. As eggs begin to set, gently pull them across the pan with a spatula. As they form large, soft lumps, continue pulling, lifting and folding until thickened, but don't stir constantly. Serve immediately once no liquid remains, over toast.

## Pumpkin risotto

*Serves 4*

Splash of olive oil
500g pumpkin, peeled and diced
½ teaspoon hot mustard powder
2 tablespoons olive oil
1 onion, finely chopped
280g arborio rice
1L vegetable or chicken stock, or broth
Salt to taste
60g grated Parmesan cheese

**METHOD**

Heat the oil in a frying pan over medium heat and add the pumpkin, tossing it so each side gleams with oil. Let it brown on each side. Tap the mustard powder through a fine sieve to dust the pumpkin on all sides. Cover and keep warm.

Heat the oil in a large saucepan over a medium-low heat and brown the onion. Turn the heat down and cook the onion gently till it's translucent and soft. Strain the oil into a bowl and keep the onion for another dish. Spatula the oil back into the pot and warm over medium-low heat.

Add the rice and stir until white spots appear in the grains, about 1 minute. Begin adding one ladleful of stock at a time, maintaining a simmer, and cook, stirring constantly, until liquid is absorbed. Continue adding and stirring until the mixture is creamy and the rice is just tender but slightly firm in the middle, about 25 minutes.

Add the Parmesan cheese, salt to taste and stir well, then mix in the pumpkin. Serve in warmed bowls.

**Other ideas:**

◆ pancakes

◆ banana custard

◆ pan-fried salmon with mashed potato

◆ tuna sandwich on white bread

# ACKNOWLEDGMENTS

We're indebted to the wonderful team at Wilkinson Publishing who have supported the project as it evolved throughout seven years of writing.

Thank you to Michael Wilkinson for giving Tim the opportunity as a previously unpublished author to write this book, and for his great patience and forbearance about the amount of time it has taken to come to fruition. Many thanks also to Jess Lomas for her capable project management and sensitive editing, and Alicia Freile at Tango Media for a magnificent cover and beautiful internal design.

We're grateful to those who generously gave their expertise and helped us get the facts right: Professor David Bowtell, Professor Jonathan Cebon, Professor Steve Ellen, Dr Sarah Francis, Erin Laing, Dr Nils Lonberg and Alexandra Stewart. And Tim would like to express his gratitude to Assistant Professor Caroline Owen for opening a number of doors to experts at the Peter MacCallum Cancer Centre.

Huge thanks to those who generously shared their stories for our case studies over the seven years it has taken to bring this book to life: Alison Jones, Louisa Pennell, Bruce Robertson, Alistair Urquhart, and those whose names have been changed for privacy reasons.

Tim would like to thank every single researcher and medical professional whose work is referred to in this book, and beyond, for what they are doing to help fewer families suffer the helplessness that he had to endure upon his father's diagnosis. And thank you to Lizzie for initial encouragement and ongoing support that has helped him get across the line.

Jackey would like to thank all the health professionals who do their utmost to keep so many of us free of cancer. And Jules, for listening.

# ABOUT THE AUTHORS

## Tim Ladhams

Tim Ladhams is the editor of *Inside Small Business* and is responsible for all the publication's online content and its quarterly magazine. He turned to journalism after a long career—including management roles—in hospitality, insurance and credit management.

Born and brought up in the United Kingdom, Tim moved to Australia in 2008 and recently moved from Melbourne to the Grampians in regional Australia. He was driven to researching the themes in this book after losing his father to cancer soon after coming to Australia.

## Jackey Coyle

Jackey Coyle is a writer, researcher and editor who has written about health and wellbeing since 2001. She is the author of *In the End: A practical guide to dying* (2021).

With her mother a nurse and her father a physicist, Jackey was immersed in medicine and science from her earliest days. She regularly practises yoga, meditation and qi gong while maintaining a long-time interest in consciousness and evidence-based holistic medicine.

Jackey lives in inner Melbourne with her husband and their extensive library of books, music and film.

Find out more about Jackey at wordygurdy.com.au.

# REFERENCES

## PROLOGUE

13      Australia consistently figures in the top countries: information was
        sourced from weforum.org

13      Australia's policy and planning infrastructure: information was sourced
        from www.brit-med.com

## CHAPTER 1: THE WORLD'S BIGGEST PROBLEM

15      global cancer deaths 2020: information was sourced from who.int/
        news-room

15      19 million cases: information was sourced from
        acsjournals.onlinelibrary.wiley.com

15      incidence in next two decades: information was sourced from gco.iarc.fr

15      cancer's total economic cost: information was sourced from who.int

16      US expenditure on cancer research: information was sourced from
        cancer.gov

16      cancer research UK: information was sourced from cancerresearchuk.org

16      cost to Australian healthcare system: information was sourced from
        cancercouncil.com.au

16      developing countries: information was sourced from who.int

16–17   cancer: definitions were sourced from cancer.gov, medicalnewstoday.com
        and canceraustralia.gov.au

19      cancer across the millennia: information was sourced from cancer.org

21      UK genome mapping project: information was sourced from
        genomicsengland.co.uk

21      immunotherapy 2013 breakthrough: information was sourced from
        cancerresearch.org

21      UCLA non-small cell lung cancer study: information was sourced from
        newsroom.ucla.edu


## CHAPTER 2: DIAGNOSTIC TECHNIQUES

26      CT scans: information was sourced from healthline.com

27      PET imaging: information was sourced from petermac.org

28      global cancer new cases: information was sourced from who.int/cancer

29      breast cancer diagnostics: information was sourced from ncri.org.uk

30      PC3A test for prostate cancer: information was sourced from
        about-cancer.cancerresearchuk.org

31      fallopian tube lavage: information was sourced from cancer.org

32      VOCs released on our breath: information was sourced from
        edition.cnn.com

32      Johns Hopkins University cancer blood test: information was sourced
        from hopkinsmedicine.org


## CHAPTER 3: SURGICAL TECHNIQUES

37–41   types of surgery: information was sourced from mdanderson.org

39      curative surgery: information was sourced from training.seer.cancer.gov

39–43   various types of surgery : information was sourced from mayoclinic.org

42      endoscopic surgery: information was sourced from cancer.org

44      electrosurgery: information was sourced from hopkinsmedicine.org/

45–7    robotic surgery: information was sourced from hopkinsmedicine.org and
        nyulangone.org

46      prostatectomy: information was sourced from prostates.com.au

46      worldwide robotic surgery event: broadcast from wrse24.org

47      pelvic organ removal: information was sourced from
        buildingbetterhealthcare.com

47      Nanoknife technology: information was sourced from
        osfhealthcare.org/blog

73      Cetuximab and Afatinib: information was sourced from cancerresearchuk.org

73      SERMs: information was sourced from breastcancer.org

74      aromatase inhibitors as a preventative: information was sourced from cancer.org

75      anti ADT-resistant drugs (prostate cancer): information was sourced from cancer.org

76      MIT mitosis study: information was sourced from news.mit.edu

78      University of Helsinki nanomedicine study: information was sourced from goodnewsfinland.com

## CHAPTER 6: IMMUNOTHERAPY

83      a paradigm shift: information was sourced from science.org

84      history of immunotherapy: information was sourced from nature.com

84      Macfarlane Burnet: information was sourced from aai.org

86      adoptive cell transfer: definition was sourced from cancer.gov

89      monoclonal antibodies: information was sourced from health.gov.au

91      Jim Allison CTLA-4 discovery: information was sourced from mdanderson.org

## CHAPTER 7: COMBINATION TREATMENTS

98      HIPEC: information was sourced from cancercenter.com

99      IORT: information was sourced from petermac.org

100     intraperitoneal chemotherapy: information was sourced from oncolink.org

100     combining chemo- and radiotherapies (SABR): information was sourced from onclive.com

102     BEP: information was sourced from macmillan.org.uk

103     advanced melanoma study: information was sourced from ncbi.nlm.nih.gov

103     Rush University Medical Centre study: information was sourced from onclive.com

104     IAP proteins: information was sourced from ncbi.nlm.nih.gov and cancerres.aacrjournals.org

## CHAPTER 8: PERSONALISED MEDICINE AND CANCER GENOMICS

106     personalised medicine: definition was sourced from cancerresearchuk.org

106     cancer genomics: definition was sourced from melbournegenomics.org.au

117     APL treatment: information was sourced from cancer.org

118     KRAS mutations: information was sourced from mdanderson.org

119     Professor Peter Johnson: information was sourced from news. cancerresearchuk.org

## CHAPTER 9: CLINICAL TRIALS

124     trial funding, Robyn Ward: information was sourced from australianclinicaltrials.gov.au

127–9   clinical trial background: information was sourced from cancer.org

132     immunotherapy timeline: information was sourced from whatisbiotechnology.org

## CHAPTER 10: PSYCHOSOCIAL ONCOLOGY

141     psychosocial oncology works: National Breast Cancer Centre, 'Clinical practice guidelines for the psychosocial care of adults with cancer', canceraustralia.gov.au, 2003

142     emotional roller-coaster: BH Fox, 'The role of psychological factors in cancer incidence and prognosis', *Oncology*, 9(3), 245: 53, 1995

143     five stages of grief: Elisabeth Kübler-Ross, *On Death and Dying*, Macmillan 1969

146     quicker recovery: Linda E Carlson and Barry D Bultz, 'Benefits of psychosocial oncology care: Improved quality of life and medical cost offset', *Health and Quality of Life Outcomes*, 1: 8, 2003

146     significant psychological distress: Stuart J Lee et al., 'Routine screening for psychological distress on an Australian inpatient haematology and oncology ward: impact on use of psychosocial services', supplement, *Medical Journal of Australia*, vol. 193, no. 5, mja.com.au, 6 September 2010

147     pilot study at The Alfred: Stuart J Lee et al., 'Routine screening for psychological distress on an Australian inpatient haematology and oncology ward: impact on use of psychosocial services', *Medical Journal of Australia*, mja.com.au, 2010

148     survivorship: Neil K Aaronson et al., 'Beyond treatment: Psychosocial and behavioural issues in cancer survivorship research and practice', *European Journal of Cancer Supplements*, vol. 12, issue 1, 2014

148     we can respond to adversity in four ways: Scott Barry Kaufman, 'Post-traumatic growth: finding meaning and creativity in adversity', *Scientific American*, blogs.scientificamerican.com/beautiful-minds/post-traumatic-growth-finding-meaning-and-creativity-in-adversity, 20 April 2020

## CHAPTER 11: LIVING WITH CANCER

152     up to 80% of people become malnourished: Alexandra Stewart, centreforcancernutrition.com

153     getting enough sleep: information was sourced from healthysleep.med.harvard.edu

154–60  nutrition content was reviewed by Erin Laing, Accredited Practising Dietitian

155     single go-to dairy source: Matthew Solan, 'Dairy: Health food or health risk?', *Harvard Health Publishing*, health.harvard.edu, 25 January 2019

157     obesity, an important risk factor: Cancer Council, 'Does sugar cause cancer?', cancer.org.au

158     sugars that break down slowly: Cassandra Szoeke, *Secrets of Women's Healthy Ageing*, Melbourne University Press, 2021

160     exercise can increase life span: Cassandra Szoeke, *Secrets of Women's Healthy Ageing*, also health.harvard.edu

160     exercise reduces cancer risk: information was sourced from blog.dana-farber.org

161     exercise creates a cancer-suppressive environment: Kim, Jin-Soo et al., 'Myokine expression and tumor-suppressive effect of serum following 12 weeks of exercise in prostate cancer patients on ADT', *Medicine & Science in Sports & Exercise*, 20 September 2021

161     effects of toxic drugs on the cardiovascular system: André La Gerche et al., 'The effect of chemotherapy on aerobic power and cardiac function in early-stage breast cancer patients', acra.net.au, 2017

161     no evidence of heart damage: SBS News, 'Exercise shown to help prevent effects of toxic drugs during cancer treatment', 27 February 2018

161–2   types of exercise and safety tips: information was sourced from cancervic.org.au

162     two-thirds of adults: Matthew Walker, *Why We Sleep: The new science of sleep and dreams*, Penguin Random House UK, 2018

163     effects of sleep deprivation: Michael R Irwin et al., 'Partial night sleep deprivation reduces natural killer and cellular immune responses in humans', *FASEB Journal* 10(5):643-53, DOI: 10.1096/fasebj.10.5.8621064, May 1996

164     medications: Matthew Walker, *Why We Sleep: The new science of sleep and dreams*, Penguin, 2018

164     a useful resource: sleephealthfoundation.org.au

164     complementary medicine evidence: Linda E Carlson et al., 'Mind-body therapies in cancer: what is the latest evidence?', pubmed.ncbi.nlm.nih.gov/28822063/, 18 August 2017

165–6   complementary therapies: information was sourced from cancervic.org.au

167     tempting with taste and smell: Alexandra Stewart, personal communication, 12 October 2021

169     surviving cancer: Australian Institute of Health and Welfare, *Cancer in Australia: In brief 2019*, Cancer series no. 122, cat no. CAN 126, Canberra: AIHW, 2019

169     2020 figures: information was sourced from cancer.org.au

170     managing cancer pain: Professor Melanie Lovell quoted in 'Media Release: The how-to expert guide for people living with cancer to help them take charge of pain', HammondCare, 27 May 2021

171     alcohol-related cancer: information was sourced from cancer.org.au